MOBILITY
FOR LIFE

MOBILITY
FOR LIFE

Healthy Joints, Strong Bones,
and a Peaceful Mind with
AVITA YOGA

JEFF BAILEY

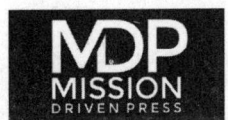

Mobility for Life: Healthy Joints, Strong Bones, and a Peaceful Mind with Avita Yoga®
Copyright © 2025 by Jeff Bailey

All rights reserved. No part of this publication may be reproduced, stored in a retrieval system, or transmitted in any form by any means, electronic, mechanical, photocopy, recording, or otherwise, without the prior permission of the publisher, except as provided by USA copyright law.

No patent liability is assumed with respect to the use of the information contained herein. Although every precaution has been taken in the preparation of this book, the publisher and author assume no responsibility for errors or omissions. Neither is any liability assumed for damages resulting from the use of the information contained herein.

This book is intended for informational purposes only. It is not intended to be used as the sole basis for medical or health decisions, nor should it be construed as advice designed to meet the particular needs of an individual's situation.

Please consult your doctor before undertaking any of the recommendations in this book, which is inspired by personal experience, observed results, and feedback from countless Avita Yoga practitioners. The information provided in this book is intended for educational and informational purposes only and should not be considered as medical advice. Yoga can involve physical exertion and carries inherent risks, including injury. By engaging in the practices outlined in this book, you acknowledge and accept that you are doing so at your own risk. The author and publisher disclaim any liability for injuries or damages arising from your use of this material. It is advisable to consult a healthcare professional before starting any new exercise program, especially if you have preexisting health conditions or concerns.

AVITA YOGA and AVITA are registered trademarks of Yoga Kaala, LLC.

Published by Mission Driven Press, an imprint of Forefront Books, Nashville, Tennessee.
Distributed by Simon & Schuster.

Library of Congress Control Number: 2025907304
Print ISBN: 978-1-63763-433-2
E-book ISBN: 978-1-63763-434-9

Cover Design by Bruce Gore, Gore Studio, Inc.
Interior Design by PerfecType, Nashville, TN

Printed in the United States of America

25 26 27 28 29 30 LSC 10 9 8 7 6 5 4 3 2 1

This book is dedicated to the students who have taught me so much.

CONTENTS

Introduction	13
Chapter 1: What Is Avita Yoga?	21
Chapter 2: Purpose Is Everything	25
The Primary Pattern	26
The Primary Goal	28
Movement Is Not Enough	29
It's Not a Balancing Act	32
Protection, Pain, and Comfort	35
You Cannot Protect Your Way into Better Health	38
A Brief History of Pain	39
The Disorganized Body	42
The Organized Body	45
Chapter 3: It's All About the Feedback	47
Immediate Feedback	49
Delayed Feedback	52
Muscle Cramps—Friend or Foe?	54
Don't Shoot the Messenger	56
Healing Sensation	57
Bones Love Pressure	59
The Sensation of Tightness	63

    The Sensation of No Sensation   64
    The Sensation of Weakness   65
    Feedback—From the Mat to Life   67
    Don't Eliminate the Sensation   68

Chapter 4: Our Trepidation with Joints   69
    Ligaments, Tendons, Muscles, and Bones   69
    Synovial Joints—The Target   71
    Gravity, Pressure, and the Lack Thereof   73
    Bones and Joints Can Be Remodeled   74
    Synovial Fluid: Joint Lubricant   76
    Metabolism, Energy, and Waste Byproducts   77
    Arthritis   80
    Fibromyalgia   84
    Other Factors Affecting Joint Health and Mobility   85

Chapter 5: Protocol for Joint Replacement   87
    Compensatory Patterns and Joint Replacements   87
    Decision-Making—To Replace or Not   90
    Prehab Before Rehab   92

Chapter 6: The Spine   95
    Fusion and Stenosis   95
    The "Dark Side of the Moon"   97

Chapter 7: Our Concern for Bones   99
    Osteoporosis and Osteopenia   99

Chapter 8: Our Fascination with Muscles   103
    We Love Them   104
    We Blame Them   106
    Size Matters Not   107
    The Four Muscle Characteristics   109
    Muscles Don't Stretch   111

Risks of Too Much "Stretch" ... 112
Wear, Tear, and Time ... 115
Flexibility vs. Mobility ... 116
The Science of "The Stretch" ... 119
Muscle and Joint Personalities ... 121

Chapter 9: Our Unawareness of the Nervous System ... 123
Neuroplasticity ... 125
A Mobile Foundation ... 127

Chapter 10: Our Ignorance with Connective Tissue ... 129
Cartilage—Preferable, but Overrated ... 133

Chapter 11: Exercise Redefined ... 135
The Need to Maintain What You Gain ... 136
Health or Fitness—Which Do You Want? ... 137
The Problem with Doing to Get ... 140

Chapter 12: The Cycle of Pain ... 143
Fix-it Mode ... 145
Posture ... 147
Compensation Patterns ... 150
Restrictions, Blockages, and Adhesions ... 152

Chapter 13: The Cycle of Healing ... 155
Resolving Chronic Pain ... 156
Healing Mode ... 157
Injury: A Healing Perspective ... 158

Chapter 14: Physical Practice ... 161
What? No Mirrors? ... 162
Levels of Practice ... 163
Featured Workshops ... 166
Practice Materials ... 166
How Often? A Little Can Be a Lot ... 168

How Much? Less Is More	169
Ready to Get Started?	171

Chapter 15: Avita Shapes and Movements — 173

Chapter 16: Results of Practice — 215
Improved Mobility	215
Better Circulation	215
A Better Walk	216
A Better Seat	216
Better Balance	216
A Better Reach	217
Better Sleep	217
A Peaceful Presence	217

Chapter 17: Quiet Breath, Quiet Mind — 219

Chapter 18: Food for Thought — 225
Meet George Jetson	226
Enjoy Real Food and Clean Water	228
Avoid Chemicals	229
Limit Sugar Consumption	230
Beware "Low Sugar" or "Zero Calories"	231
Watch Out for Plant-Based Fats and Oils	232
Go Beyond the Label	233
Minimize Processed Foods	233
Go Organic and Non-GMO	234
Enjoy the Fat with the Protein	234
Nourish Your Gut	235
Skip a Meal	237

Chapter 19: Know Your Constitution — 239
The Flexible Constitution—"I Want to Feel My Body"	240
The Rigid Constitution—"I'm Not Flexible Enough"	241
The Athletic Constitution—"I Can Do Anything"	242

Putting It All Together—"I Want Peace of Mind"   243

Chapter 20: Know Your Inner Rhythm   245
    Namaste   247

Acknowledgments   249
Notes   251
About the Author   259

INTRODUCTION

Life happens, and then somewhere along the way, it catches up to us, and we find that our body doesn't function with the same ease that it did in our youth. Nobody can avoid the effects of time and gravity and various traumas that occur over a lifetime. I'm no exception. I am not an inherently flexible person. My gains have come by experimenting with my body and turning injuries and setbacks into healing opportunities. I have opened my heart to the classroom of life, and it has shown me a revolutionary way to peace, health, and mobility. This book aims to convey my discoveries so that you may live more comfortably and fully in your body.

Many will agree that yoga has a component that goes beyond stretching the body. For me, the real changes have come with stretching my mind. In Avita, we don't stretch or push the body at all. As you will learn, it's not so much what we do but *how* we do it.

At the age of twenty-two, I fell in love with the physical and spiritual practice of yoga. Decades later, I found myself searching for ways to recover from a ski accident that severely impacted my hip. The yoga, the PT, the massage, the exercises—none of them would relieve the pain, and at the young age of fifty-one, a doctor told me that a hip replacement was in my future. This book is a result of my determination to find a better way.

Unbeknownst to me at the time, yoga would become a means to heal my mind. It was the summer of 1985, and yoga breathed fresh air into my life. It got my attention, and something inside said, *Stay with this. There is an ocean of knowledge waiting for you.* Heartfelt intuition speaks to us soft and whisper-like, an inner tickle. The seed was planted, and after my first class, I asked the teacher, Dr. Norman Allard, "What is yoga?" He said it means "to join." I thought to myself, *That's odd. If yoga means "to join," why do we spend so much time pulling ourselves apart?* For me, the definition did not match the practice. And there began my spiritual journey. Only later did I realize the power and importance of the question, "What does it mean to join?" Most people equate yoga with stretching and the belief that you must be flexible to do it. Many feel that if they can't, they shouldn't. But what good is that? If yoga means "to join," what's missing in our interpretation? Shouldn't joining be something everyone can do?

Our childhood roots play a requisite and often unpredictable role in future endeavors. The son of a veterinarian, I grew up on a small ranch in rural Gunnison, Colorado, where work and play were synonymous. I enjoyed my responsibilities, loved the land, appreciated the local people, and developed an affinity for looking after small and large animals.

Whether it was a cow, a calf, or a fence, it had to be tended and mended. I had my hands on everything. I assisted with countless surgeries and saw the inner workings of many different animals. I felt moving lungs and beating hearts, sometimes as life left the body. I watched in awe once as my dad performed CPR on a colt, slamming his body weight into its chest, giving it mouth-to-nostril resuscitation, and bringing it back to life. I watched him stitch torn muscle tissue and pin bones back together in dogs and cats that were hit by cars. I assisted with so many spays that I begged him to switch roles with me, but for obvious reasons, he never obliged. I learned firsthand how fragile bodies are and saw life come and go regularly. These were the years I learned to care.

At some point in our journey, we realize there are no mistakes. There may be injuries, but no mistakes. *Everything* is perfectly designed to help us awaken and heal if we allow ourselves to be truly helpful—a perspective that also brings purpose to all we do.

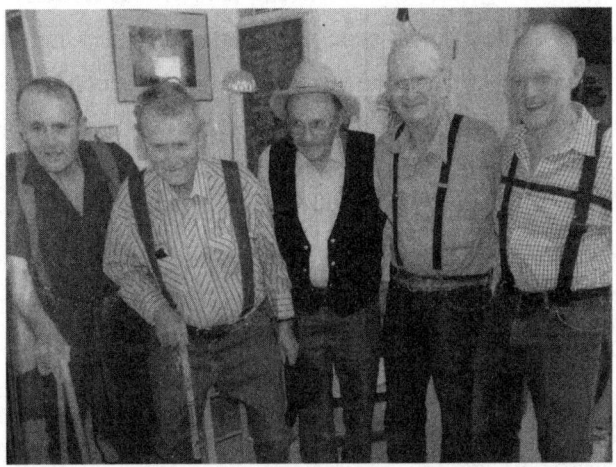

I adored my uncles and my dear dad. They had an uncanny sense of humor, probably necessary to get them through life's challenges. They, especially my dad (on the right), inspired me in countless ways.

I never imagined my life would revolve around yoga, but looking back, I could not have asked for a better foundation for a career in yoga. My childhood was the perfect backdrop that led to the circumstances, insights, and creation of Avita Yoga. Watching the effects of time and gravity on my uncles and dad inspired me to find a way to stay upright and mobile. I developed an excellent understanding of anatomy and physiology at an impressionable age, but inner guidance would not let me pursue a medical degree. I wanted to preserve my autonomy and felt my education and life function would be found outside of the medical world. Integrating yoga with the body's healing physiology and the mind's unlimited curative power has been a lifetime of joyous work.

In the early 1990s, a knee injury led me to discover, benefit from, and train to become a certified Rolfer™. The training was life-changing and set me on a course for Avita Yoga. It was fascinating to learn in the shadows of a pioneer like the late Ida Rolf, PhD, and see how injury, gravity, and psychology impact the human body—how it can become structurally disorganized over time.[1] I learned how the caring use of hands, fingers, thumbs, and elbows could reorganize the body's connective tissues and help it become more structurally integrated. I learned to recognize bodily disorganization, identify unhealthy movement patterns, and see the parts that lack healthy movement. I soon realized you can't just "do yoga" or stretch your way into better structure, because we unwittingly move in the patterns we're trying to resolve. The restrictions and patterns follow us until we isolate and *undo* them. An organized body functions better in countless ways. Additionally, Rolfing Movement® was a way to further develop hands-on work and see the results through a movement-reeducation process. Along the journey I learned how to empower clients to own and incorporate these positive results into their lives.

This chapter of my life profoundly impacted me and reshaped my understanding of yoga. I discovered that when I worked on people in a specific yoga shape, the results would come quicker and last longer. It worked even better for those willing to practice a few suggested yoga shapes at home or attend the twice-weekly yoga classes I taught out of the old Rolf Institute® at 302 Pearl in Boulder. It was during these years between 1994 and 1999 that I realized I enjoyed teaching and had developed a knack for reducing complex ideas to simple, understandable terms.

In 2009, a series of harrowing personal losses humbled me to my knees. Ego-pride had taken over, and everything that had seemed to go my way was suddenly turned upside down. The inner pain was so profound that no outer help could touch it. And so, for the first time, I prayed at an equally deep level.

Help came in the form of small but meaningful turnarounds, and in the fall of 2010, the answer I needed arrived through a dream that blew my heart open. It felt like a direct experience with perfect Universal Love. Everything changed, and as problems became opportunities to heal, they disappeared. I perceived the world in a whole new way. I heard a new and loving inner Voice saying, *Write*. I listened and followed.

I wrote every day as healing thoughts of universal truth poured through. I would sit with my friend Gene Langlois weekly to share and refine the words. In March 2014, we published *The Yoga Mind: The Yoga Sutras According to a Course in Miracles*.

Two years earlier, driving south on Broadway in Boulder, my wife, Lori, had broken the silence with a question. "If a place in south Boulder were available to open a yoga studio, would you want to?" I quickly scanned south Boulder in my mind, determined that no such place existed, and replied, "Yes." Say yes to the universe, and it *will* respond, and sure enough, days later, Lori found what became Yoga Loft, a most beautiful yoga studio with amazing views of Boulder's Flatirons. Then she found us a partner, Nikki Rogers, who was immensely helpful in launching the business and later sold her ownership back to us. I am forever grateful for Nikki.

I perceived the yoga industry then as a motorboat speeding through the water, leaving disenchanted and sometimes injured students in its wake. Yoga Loft Boulder and the yoga I would teach was for those in the wake—those who were injured from yoga and those who believe flexibility is a requirement to practice. We wanted to create a non-competitive environment where everyone felt welcome no matter what their body type, size, or attire. With pure faith, we opened the doors in the fall of 2012. The classroom of life took me deeper still.

One beautiful winter day on Vail Mountain, I was having the time of my life skiing with my good friend Philippe. Making fast giant-slalom (GS) turns, our hips collided at the apex of a turn, because we were in each other's blind spot. Our gear was scattered everywhere. Dizzy and humbled, we picked up the pieces and called it a day.

The real pain came a few days later. I began to limp, and I developed sciatic nerve pain that I could not shake. For the first time in years, the yoga I was doing did not solve my problem. PT didn't work, and the orthopedic doctors told me it would get worse and eventually lead to a hip replacement. I took the information in but didn't let it land on my heart. What I had to do *now* was find a way to solve the pain. Months went by. It was not easy, but it gave me time to forgive myself for the accident, which, despite the annoying pain, allowed the Voice for Reason to come through. I was reminded that nothing happens by chance.

Resting on my back after yoga one day, I willed for a better way. I closed my eyes, and without attachment, I sincerely asked for a way to resolve my hip pain and fulfill my vision of providing a style of yoga that would benefit those who can't "do yoga."

A week or two later, I found myself in a yoga class, in a position that put pressure on the traumatized area of my hip, and I knew this was going to resolve my hip problem and pain. I realized the healing potency of following the pain and slowly adding pressure. Intuitive guidance that had brought me this far told me yoga needed to evolve and be shared. I didn't need to nor want to do the hard work of forming a new yoga brand. However, the yet unrealized healing potential of what I knew yoga could become inspired me. I could not ignore the call. Avita Yoga was born.

Avita's philosophy and purpose of practice differ from *all* forms of yoga and that will come through as you read this book. Even so, it does not matter what form of yoga you are drawn to, but it *is* essential to look carefully at the purpose you give it. Purpose is given, not found. And with a bit of quiet reflection, you will find that purpose is our only real choice in all we do—to *heal* or not. *To join* or uphold a sense of separate self. Shakespeare distilled the pain of the human condition and the illusion that death would resolve it into one crucial question we can apply to any moment: To *be* or not to be.[2]

This practice called Avita Yoga came *to* me and then *through* me as a means to heal, learn, and share our universal truth. It all began to add up: the time with my dad, the early days of yoga, and questioning its definition. Thirty-plus years with *A Course in Miracles* and the experience of lasting peace and happiness it promises formed the foundation of my life, our marriage, and my yoga. As a graduate student, I learned conflict resolution skills and group leadership as an Outward Bound instructor. My Rolfing® certification was the best yoga teacher training I ever had, and insights from the Yoga Sutras and the experience of writing my first book, *The Yoga Mind*, deepened my spiritual foundation. Always a student, I had many teachers contribute to Avita, making it a culmination of a life dedicated to a desire to be truly helpful. Methodologies were discarded if they didn't fit Love's heartfelt Guidance. Life *is* the path. It will lead us to the peaceful truth within if we let it.

Neither lineage nor legacy are important. One looks backward and the other looks forward, but they are both rooted in the past. Neither lasts and valuing either keeps us out of the present moment. The question is, does whatever is "left behind" unify or promote specialness and separation? It's our yoga to heal and to heal is to join. The decision is yours. Like my friend Gene would often say, the truth is true because it is changeless, formless, perfect, and eternal.

Avita evolves as I evolve, but the founding principles remain unchanged because they follow a direct and timeless formula: Don't seek for truth but rather identify and resolve the barriers to it. This is how we heal, join, and let intuitive Guidance come through.

Avita Yoga is a gem that has restored my sense of youth and radically changed how I see health, fitness, and our potential to heal. In many ways, an Avita practice can reverse the aging process in body and mind. When we feel younger in our bones, we become more youthful and welcome spontaneity into our lives. And when something works, we naturally want to share it, which is why this book is in your hands.

At some point along the way, I realized the yoga needed a name that goes beyond Jeff Bailey. Lori and I went through hundreds of possibilities and many doodled pieces of paper. I often found names I liked and translated them into Sanskrit, but they would sometimes be hard to pronounce or spell. Among the themes for practice was "yoga for life," which became the tagline and now part of the title for this book. And that's how Avita came through: The Latin root of the word means "for life."

CHAPTER 1

What Is Avita Yoga?

Countless methods and exercises will strengthen muscles to protect and stabilize joints, but none directly fortify the joints. We understand exercise, but there is no paradigm for a program specifically for joint and bone health, which is why it takes an entire book to bend the mind in a new and different way. This book aims to explain, motivate, and move the needle toward a revolutionary approach to joint health and lasting mobility that can save energy, money, and time. That said, you need not finish the book to begin practice! I've found definitions of Avita to be lifeless compared to the *experience* of practice. Find an Avita teacher near you, or join me online at www.AvitaYogaOnline.com and practice as you read.

When our joints are in pain and call for attention, we typically target the muscles to fortify or support the joint, which can miss the problem. No one gets muscle replacements. It's the joints that are signaling for help! Still, we strengthen and stretch the muscles and someday wonder why we need surgery or joint replacements.

So, how do we target the joints? Thoughtfully and sustainably. Later, you will read about your inherent healing physiology that cleanses and remodels your bones and joints (chapter 4). Avita movements and the compression they generate stimulate this healing process within the joint. The result is improved mobility and diminished pain; the good news is that it takes less time to dissolve blockages than you might think.

Avita is not the yoga popularized through fitness trends, athleticism, and the goal of a better look. Instead, Avita acknowledges the limits and barriers in the body and resolves them. We skip no steps as we aim to increase circulation, diminish pain and increase the chances for mobility for life. We do not push the body or the form. We let the yoga come to us.

Why subvert the healing power of *now* with the false notion that accomplishing the "pose" will bring future results? We cannot push our bodies to extremes and obtain healthy long-term results. In my lifetime, I've seen yoga and fitness trends become *increasingly creatively intense*. We're attracted to the extreme imagery for the health and happiness it symbolizes. Many are drawn to these demanding forms of fitness but are soon disenchanted and stop. Avita is for those who want an accessible approach to sustainable results.

It's been valuable for me to question yoga trends that aim to align body parts for an outer achievement or look. Unlike "poses," Avita uses *shapes* to find blockages to mobility, restore joint health, and increase bone density. It's a slow, deep approach. Perfecting a *pose* depends on outer evaluation. Perfecting an *experience* relies on a relationship with yourself. Which do you listen to and follow: a judgment or a heartfelt feeling? Avita Yoga is an inside job—an inner inquiry.

Avita identifies and removes obstacles to mobility while fostering a deep sense of inner peace. We are far less concerned about flexibility in Avita because *mobility* is found in the joints, and *flexibility* has more to do with body types. Your joints and bones love steady compression, and a little goes a long way. The shapes and movements bring them healing pressure. We don't stretch. Avita uses kind, compressive forces to dissolve the restrictions to improve mobility, cleanse joints, and strengthen bones while learning to be peaceful and present.

Often attributed to Rumi, there are two timeless sentences from *A Course in Miracles* that guide my yoga and my life: "Your task is not to seek for love, but merely to seek and find all of the barriers within yourself that you have built against it. It is not necessary to seek for what is true, but it *is* necessary to seek for what is false."[3] It is a timeless formula that consistently works for those who want true love. Notice how beautifully it translates to life: Your yoga is not to seek mobility but to seek, find, and resolve the barriers to mobility. The dissolution of restrictions is very different than trying to attain mobility. Want better balance? A better walk? Better health? Remove the barriers to them and they are yours.

Avita is thus an undoing. We *do* to *undo*. It's the Zen nature of practice. How can I "do" the practice to *un*do the barriers to my desired freedom? We will only find the answer through experience, for words alone are insufficient. "Undoing" must originate in the mind because it requires a forgiving approach.

By removing the barriers to love and the barriers to mobility, I have personally found more peace and more freedom, and I have witnessed it in countless others. Thank you for joining me on this healing inner journey with Avita Yoga.

CHAPTER 2

Purpose Is Everything

Yoga must have a higher purpose, for physical exertion or advancement alone will not lead to a lasting sense of unity and wholeness. A better body alone is the wrong goal. Sweat may cleanse the body, but it won't bring lasting happiness and peace. With a gentle change in perspective, we realize that favorable outcomes reflect the more profound inner work and a desire to heal.

Remember the Star Wars scene where Luke Skywalker became frustrated trying to raise the spaceship from the water? Remember Yoda's timeless words? "No. Try not. Do or do not. There is no try."[4] When the words finally sank into Luke's heart and mind, he didn't work harder. He didn't try harder. He let go. He let go of his self-pity and joined The Force by releasing his fear and disbelief.

As a willing student, can you begin to accept your body exactly as it is? Yes? Then, could you bring it to your practice without demanding a predetermined change? Can you give it the opportunity to heal in the present by releasing the past? We've all experienced trauma to varying degrees , but now is the time to let it go. Until we forgive our past, it goes with us everywhere we go. Whether you are conscious of it or not, Avita shapes bring the past to the healing light of now. We practice and get on with our day by kindly putting one foot in front of the other with more freedom in each step.

THE PRIMARY PATTERN

Time erodes, and gravity collapses. This primary pattern is the result of time and gravity on the body. It usually shows up later in life but starts earlier than we think. Throw in a few social or familial rules and impositions on the body, and you have a recipe for problems. You've seen it in others; perhaps you've noticed it in yourself. If there were a way to identify and resolve this pattern and the restrictions that maintain it, would you want to know about it?

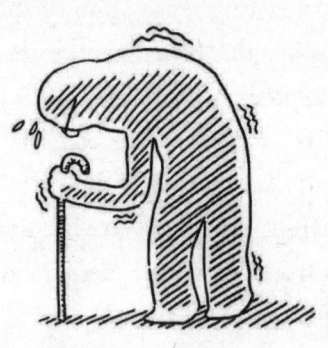

Let's dig deeper into the primary pattern to give us insights into its undoing. Here's what happens on our journey through time, gravity, and form. The knees begin to buckle, and the feet get rigid. The front part of the hip becomes shortened and stuck. The lower part of the back stiffens, and the upper back tends to round and hunch forward. Shoulder movement is restricted, and reaching overhead gets harder. The head and neck can accommodate the rest of the body's patterns in many ways, but they mostly posture forward. Essentially, the front of the body gets shorter, ankles stiffen, knees buckle, and the back struggles to stay upright.

Routine activities like putting a shirt on or reaching for a mug on the top shelf become more difficult and eventually impossible. As the hip and lower back become rigid, lifting each leg to negotiate stairs becomes increasingly tricky. Washing our feet, pulling socks on, and tying shoes becomes more difficult. The feet, being at the bottom of the structure, collect toxins. As time goes by, toes and feet calcify, as do other joints that don't get the healthy pressure to flush and replenish the interstitial fluids in and around the joints. One reason we spend time in the practice with the legs up the wall is to challenge circulation and facilitate lymphatic flow. Hands and fingers become arthritic because we use them in the same limited way—partly because of repetitious movements but mainly because the larger primary pattern influences how we use the fingers, hands, and arms.

These degradations have become so entwined with the aging process that we plan for them. We unwittingly plan for our demise, never even suspecting there could be a better way. We know so little about aging because we tend to fight it rather than understand it. We'd sooner pop a pill or undergo surgery to keep the body going a little longer than take a holistic approach and use the symptoms to find the problem.

We go to the gym and try to exercise it all away. But we exercise *in* the primary pattern, which reinforces it. You cannot push weights around or put a demand on the body and expect it to perform outside its pattern because it *needs* the pattern to get the job done. Performance-based exercise, including some styles of yoga, not only hides the compensation patterns we're trying to resolve but reinforces them! Movement will be compromised unless we identify and target the unhealthy restrictions and the unconscious habits they foster.

This is why any helpful practice becomes an inquiry; a contemplative approach to identify and resolve limiting restrictions, thoughts, and beliefs. We avoid nothing and welcome everything, which is why our yoga is *now*. The path is gently *through*, not around.

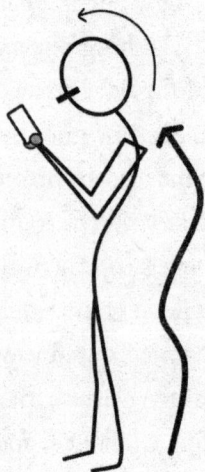

Regardless of our age, we need a way to disrupt the hidden patterns and unwind the debilitating restrictions.

The primary pattern manifests differently in each of us, but identifying it is the precursor to solving the effects of time, gravity, and a history of injuries. We don't have to analyze and understand it. We use Avita shapes to "bump into the limit" and spend time with it to unwind the primary pattern on physical and neurological levels and thus to inspire increased mobility and health.

THE PRIMARY GOAL

I know you want more comfort and less pain. I know you are concerned about your knee, hip, or shoulder and want to regain youthful movement and energy. I understand these desires, and I have them for myself. But to get the most from your practice, can you join me and reverse your thinking a bit? Beyond your pain and mobility concerns, could you let *peace of mind* be your primary goal?

Results will come faster and have more meaning if you make peace your primary goal. We resist inner peace because it seems trite and elusive, if not impossible. But please consider this helpful change in perspective: Your pain and desire to maintain mobility for life bring you to practice Avita where you learn peaceful presence. Can you sense the gentle stretch we put on the mind? Bodily perfection is not required. Plant the seed *now* and let the goal for a better body be secondary to the primary goal for peace.

Avita stimulates inner physiology to remedy and repair, and those who set the goal for peace get better and faster results. Why? Because to the mind, peace and healing are synonymous. When we drop into our joints with the desire for inner peace, health and happiness will naturally follow. The healing power of *now* is hidden when we try to change the body according to past ideals to bring a predetermined future result.

Establish peace as your primary goal, which is a practice of releasing the past and future, and healing follows. The shapes more readily dissolve the restrictions and blockages to movement. As we let go, it all becomes "small stuff." Relationships become more meaningful. We smile more often. We open up to heartfelt intuition and *follow it*. With peace as the goal, anything is possible.

With peace as the primary goal, we aim to mend joints, resolve pain, dissolve the primary pattern—the long-term effects of time and gravity on the human body. This is what makes Avita very practical. Who wouldn't want to walk through life peaceful, agile, upright, and happy?

MOVEMENT IS NOT ENOUGH

Wouldn't it be great to remain mobile and comfortable to the very end—to stay out of assisted living, shop for yourself, and get dressed on your own? That might sound funny if you're under fifty, but I cannot think of a more practical goal at any age. The problem is we believe that if we keep doing what we've always done, we'll remain able-bodied for life. Rarely does this work.

It's a mistake to assume that the movement you are doing today—whether it be walking, hiking, cycling, or working in the yard—will keep you healthy and mobile in the future.

I sometimes see people struggling to walk—some with a cane or walking stick to help them along. It is an acceptable exercise and an excellent way to enjoy the outdoors. But beneath the activity is a voice that says, *I need to keep going. If I stop moving, I'll lose my ability to move altogether.* The motivation? That movement today will ensure movement tomorrow. The problem is that we walk and exercise in the primary pattern that accommodates and reinforces the patterns contributing to the restrictions! We unwittingly move *around* the restriction, which means movement alone will not increase mobility. If we want to remain mobile and youthful for life, we need to identify and resolve the restrictions and patterns that limit us and bring pain.

Complications arise because the restricted areas often lack sensation while causing pain in other body parts. Degenerative joint disease (DJD), for example, is painless in most people as it silently develops. Like tooth decay, most don't encounter the causative culprits until pain is felt and procedures are needed.

When the pain comes, we make it a decoy and avert the causative problem. In an ongoing effort to eliminate it, we pop pills, jump into surgery, and avoid the movements that seem to cause the pain. Instead, why not find, isolate, and resolve the problem at its source? Moving, exercising, or strengthening our way out of pain brings temporary results at best, because we attempt to resolve pain while remaining in the pattern that produces the problem. These good intentions don't get to the heart of the problem, which is almost always in and around the joints, held in connective tissue, and hardwired into the nervous system.

There is a better way. We need not assume that we'll "naturally" lose mobility and independence. It doesn't have to go that way, and it helps to start sooner rather than later.

PURPOSE IS EVERYTHING

LET'S PRACTICE

Remember: Movement is not enough. We move our fingers and thumbs in many ways, yet we are unaware that arthritis could be brewing in them. Try this: Spread your fingers and thumbs wide, one hand at a time, with the palm stretching open. Hold for twenty to thirty seconds, then cross your thumb to the base of your little finger. It's the typical expression of the number four but dynamic. Can you straighten the four fingers while flexing the thumb toward the base of the pinkie? What do you feel? The work? The opposing actions, minor discomfort, or arthritic pain? What do you feel in your wrists? It's all yoga! We aim to discover the blockages and restore them to health. Hold for another minute or two, but don't push. When it's time, release slowly. Don't shake out your hand but rest it on your lap and see what you find in the other hand.

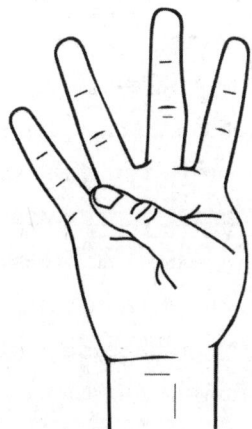

Scan the QR code to access Let's Practice video:

IT'S NOT A BALANCING ACT

Our ability to balance is primarily a function of mobility—too much or too little, and we must compensate. Other contributing factors to good balance exist, but if mobility is missing, especially in the lower body, balance will be compromised. Why do we want good balance? Simple: to keep from falling. I've seen ambitious yoga students struggle to hold the fancy poses that require balance. Often, the attention is not on the mobility necessary for balance but on holding the pose and "getting it right." We get better at what we practice. I learned that from my guitar teacher. So, rather than practicing wobbling, we practice exactly what we want and generate mobility and stability where needed to reorganize the body for healthy balance. It's not fancy but it's practical.

Rigidity shows up as a limited range of motion, which impedes our natural ability to balance, but not so obvious is how joint pain and restriction contribute to the loss of balance. Have you noticed how the smallest impulse of pain can affect your stability? The compulsion is to avoid the problem and any movement that exacerbates the pain. The onset of arthritis, tendonitis, calcification, or degeneration pushes us out of balance, into compensation patterns, and toward a false feeling of weakness. So, we go to the gym to regain strength and stamina, which can be helpful in the short term but in the long term may avoid the problematic source.

In my experience, strengthening exercises sometimes work for joint issues not because we get stronger but because the movements are focused enough and consistent enough to inadvertently bring movement and compression to the source of the problem in the connective tissues, joints, and bones. Strengthening routines may target the *muscles*, but the exercise inadvertently begins to cleanse and restore the *joints*. Avita repurposes the muscles to source the problem and the pain it generates where it can be resolved. It saves time and effort, but we don't stop the yoga just because we begin to feel better. A little preventative maintenance goes a long way.

Nothing is more disruptive to generous movement and balance than a sharp feeling of pain. Have you ever lost your balance putting your pants on because of a quick jab of pain? It can happen walking up or down stairs in our later years. It throws us out of the moment and movement, and we must stop, sit down, or quickly grab something stable to keep from falling. Don't wait for this phenomenon to occur. At some point in the aging process, walking becomes a balancing act where we have to put one foot in front of the other, maintain balance, and sometimes negotiate the pain points as we walk. It's helpful to target these painful areas with Avita as soon as you feel them. Movement is medicine and motion is lotion when we target the joints to resolve restrictions and unwind patterns that work against us.

Lastly, regarding balance, we'll focus on the important role of *feet and ankles*. More than half of the bones in your body are in your hands and feet. The fifty-two bones in your feet make up about one-quarter of all the 206 bones in your body. More bones means more movable parts to keep healthy and clean. Your entire structure balances on adaptive and mobile feet and ankles. If they are not articulating properly, your ability to balance will be limited.

But what do we do with our feet? We put them in sometimes cruelly shaped, aesthetic, protective containers that limit movement. Shoes are here to stay but have contributed to more structural problems than any other accessory. It's okay; you don't have to throw them out. Well, there might be a few that you decide to toss. Understanding what they are doing and, thus, to the rest of your body can motivate you to mobilize the bones and joints in your feet. You may also be inclined to kick your shoes off occasionally and walk barefoot.

Nothing contributes more to your ability to balance and walk than foot and ankle mobility. In many ways, we practice Avita to have a better walk. Instead of trying to improve your balance by standing on one foot, if you increase the health and mobility of your feet, knees, and hips, then your vestibular system will naturally take care of the rest.

LET'S PRACTICE

Stand facing a wall with the toes of your right foot close but not touching the baseboard and your two hands on the wall supporting you at shoulder height. Keep your eyes open and your hands on the wall. Take a fairly big step back with your left foot and place it in line with your right foot as if standing on a balance beam with both feet flat on the floor. Now, turn each heel out about an inch and feel the subtle internal rotation in each hip. Resonate with and get to know this sensation. It's healing. After about twenty seconds, use your quadriceps to straighten your knees and engage the buttocks. Keep your eyes open and move the tailbone down and the pubic bone up toward the ceiling. Refrain from overworking the shape, but feel the engagement of your musculature, squeezing the bones of your legs, knees, and hips.

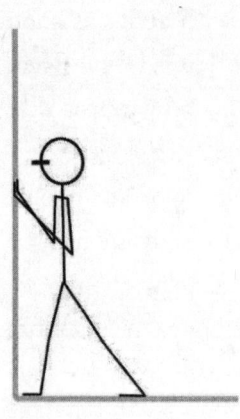

Can you sustain this shape for a minute or two? It will reveal patterns and restrictions that impede balance while fortifying your ability moment by moment. When the time is right, bend your knees, release the shape, and move the left foot to the wall, taking a big step back with the right foot, but not so big that you can't keep your heels firmly on the floor. Turn the heels out about an inch, repeat confidently as you unwind restrictions, and nurture your ability to balance. With some practice, you can sustain the shape longer and experiment with closing your eyes while keeping your hands on the wall. Because we get better at what we practice, we always practice successfully. This shape is an indicator of basic balance. The large variety of Avita shapes are all meant to mobilize joints and make this shape more doable.

Scan the QR code to access Let's Practice video:

There is an endless array of activities and methods available to keep moving and "get fit," but very few promote lasting mobility and health at the level of the bones. I've tried most, and many didn't work, but I never threw away the inspiration behind them. With Avita, we have many ways of targeting the restrictions and hidden compensation patterns in the feet, often while addressing other body parts like the knees and hips. We leave no bone out because we want every joint in the body to flex and extend fully without pain for a lifetime. Want to fortify your Avita practice with a strength program? That's fine, especially if you enjoy it. I have found that when we take care of our bones and joints, our muscles will take care of themselves.

PROTECTION, PAIN, AND COMFORT

As humans, we are programmed to avoid pain and seek comfort. On the surface, this sounds wonderful and makes perfect sense. Why would we want it any other way? And that's the critical point: We don't want it any other way until we realize the cost.

Seeking comfort keeps our mental and emotional pain hidden. Conscious of it or not, we push the pain down and cover it with compensatory thoughts and behaviors like anger, attack, projection, depression, substance abuse, and unhealthy eating. The cover-up, however, is not limited to seemingly negative behavior patterns. The discomfort can be pushed down with acceptable overtones like developing a positive attitude, "putting on a smile," and people-pleasing. These behaviors keep us stuck in the past because we're afraid of what might happen if we are more transparent and honest with ourselves and those around us. Guilt, a hideous form of self-punishment, takes over, and we keep our deepest thoughts private because we are terrified of being "found out," which makes us feel anxious and alone. When the subconscious guilt and pain become unbearable, we project them onto others, which only deepens the pain and unhealthy side effects in ourselves. Energetically, giving and receiving are the same and instantaneous. As Henry David Thoreau pointed out, the internal struggle is not obvious, and it leads to a life of "quiet desperation."

Big or small, when I attack, I suffer. When I defend, I cannot escape the effects of my own hurtful thoughts, and I avoid self-healing potential. The ego or false self uses the body for attack, pleasure, and pride.[5] The good news is that these puffs of nothingness are not our true thoughts. It's our yoga to access the underlying conditions and beliefs that foster false and limiting thoughts of fear and separation. How do we do that? We ask for help in letting the darkness come to the surface of awareness where it can be held up to the light and released. We heal by choosing to allow those limiting influences to be replaced with true thoughts of forgiveness, kindness, unity, and love. These are the thoughts of the true Self, and It *always* has our highest and best interest in mind. Think of it as heartfelt intuition. It always feels good to follow it. Even when the guidance moves us into unfamiliar territory, we can always trust this helpful inner voice.

This process takes gentle willingness to let others in and see us as we are. With great relief, we eventually let down our masks as we release our concern for the outcome. Why delay healing? It requires courage and trust to let the painful feelings, memories, and emotions surface where they can be released and resolved. No pain or problem is too big for this timeless approach to peace and happiness.

On the comfort-seeking front, humans have done a remarkable job of dodging the burdens of cohabitating with nature. Instead of adapting to the environment like other species, we alter it to fit our needs and wants. This programming runs deep—there's no changing it, and that's okay. Recognizing how it works against us, however, can be remarkably helpful.

Our ability to alter the outer for greater comfort is a perfect setup for all kinds of problems. The efficiencies and benefits of everything from smartphones to automobiles are impressive but come at a cost. The further we remove ourselves from nature, the more fragile we become. We have moved away from "natural work," where we interact with the environment. We've farmed it out! To get in touch with our roots, it can be healthy and helpful to partake in manual work whenever possible. It's good for the body and good for the mind. It's a way to reconnect with our environment and work with it rather than against it.

We're human, though, so go ahead and make the seat adjustment. Adjust the room temperature. But do the yoga to regain your adaptability. Consider a mindset that says, "I want to find the problem before it finds me." Don't have the time, you say? If you don't *make* time for healing, your body will make it for you. When we "do" our yoga and practice the shapes to reveal the problematic areas, we feel better and save time. The longer we delay, the more arduous and costly the solution becomes.

Decide there's a better way, practice, and you will see that time adjusts accordingly as you prioritize healing over tasking. You'll soon learn that pain is not the problem but a valuable messenger that can lead you to the problem so it can be resolved. This starkly contrasts with our conditioning to avoid or eliminate pain, which inadvertently protects the underlying problem and goes against the universally accepted "use it or lose it" principle.

YOU CANNOT PROTECT YOUR WAY INTO BETTER HEALTH

A brace, a crutch, and a strengthening program can certainly be helpful in rehabilitation. Do the physical therapy, but know that we cannot strengthen, protect, or preserve our way into better health. The idea that we can effectively protect ourselves is a misnomer that has elbowed its way into our lives—an unhealthy side effect of our pain-avoiding, comfort-seeking nature. In a yoga workshop, I once heard a teacher explain how he compromises his walk to find comfort in his arthritic knees. Can you see how deep pain avoidance is? Can you imagine how any compensated movement will push the problem to other areas of the body?

Prevention is one thing—protection is another. The more we protect, the more we limit mobility. It's an urge that increases as we age. We stop doing enjoyable activities, life gets narrower, and any pain sensations remind us of the need to protect, which spins us deeper into the pain cycle discussed later in the book.

Avita is a way out of pain because we don't avoid the problem. We find it. Practice prevents future joint problems and restores health to chronically affected or arthritic joints. Still, Avita does not take a protective approach. It requires a gentle paradigm shift because we won't get to the problem if we avoid the pain. We must learn to identify and question our thoughts and beliefs because many are not useful for our well-being, and may even be irrational. If you want to improve your joint health, you must question the timidity you may have with your bones and joints. Challenge the ambition to keep moving as the only way to keep moving.

Joints love pressure, but too much too fast is what we call an *injury*, and we've all experienced that. The memory of injuries makes us cautious. The older we get, the more careful we become. It's normal, and caution can go a long way, especially as we age. The question is: Will I take the familiar path to protect myself and avoid the pain? Or will I experiment with my life, kindly accept responsibility, and journey inward on the less traveled path?

With Avita, it's not only what we do but *how* we do it. Memories, feelings, and thoughts are welcome in every moment and shape. Bring your mindset to the practice. Bring your troubles, concerns, and fears. They are all part of the restriction. Listen to the cues. Avita teachers spend as much time backing students off and slowing them down as they do talking them through the shapes. We cue the same shape for everyone in the room, knowing each will have their unique version and process. We steadily unwind the patterns and problems, getting closer to the primary goal, where peace becomes our guide as we dissolve restrictions and promote restoration through the muscles, bones, and joints.

A BRIEF HISTORY OF PAIN

No pain is a poor indicator of physical health. When do you begin feeling the pain of an infected tooth? When do you feel the pain of disc or joint degeneration? Exactly: when it's too late. And so, the absence of pain can be a poor indicator of the severity of an underlying condition.

In a 2015 study, researchers compared the MRI scan results of over 3,000 people of varying ages without back pain.[6] Here's what they found:

37% of twenty-year-olds had degenerative discs. This rose to 96% in eighty-year-olds.

30% of twenty-year-olds had a disc bulge. This rose to 84% in eighty-year-olds.

There was some evidence of spinal degeneration in almost everybody.

They all showed some evidence of a condition assumed to cause pain, yet all were pain-free when the MRI was taken. Pain or not, we use the shapes to bring healing compression to the bones and joints with the goal of maintaining pain-free mobility for life.

When you stub your toe, the pain and the problem are immediate. But with chronic pain and degeneration, we usually don't know about the problem soon enough. Too often, the body pushes the issue out of awareness, and one day, out for a jog, there's an awkward step that tweaks the knee enough to bring the pain to the surface and reveal years of degeneration. Would you like to do something about it now or hope you "get lucky" and never feel the implications of degenerative joints? Teeth provide a similar example. Decay can build over many years with no pain at all, and then one day, a bite into a sandwich reveals a brewing infection and the need for a root canal. All too often my wife, the dentist, would hear something like, "But everything was fine until I bit into the sandwich."

Fortunately, the body usually sends us pain signals along the way. In the early stages, the pain often comes and goes before becoming more intense and consistent. Some ignore these early-warning signals. Some pop a pain pill. Others massage it away. Some call the doctor, while others avoid the doctor. Some react out of fear and stop the movement or activity that brings the pain. What do you do with pain signals? It's helpful to pause and ponder how you handle pain or any other "unwanted" messenger.

Symptoms are not the problem; they are the effects of a deeper cause. Treating symptoms is like cutting a weed instead of removing the root. The weed will keep coming back. In Avita, we use the symptoms to lead us to the problem where it can be resolved, and since the body remembers everything, it provides the perfect subject matter for our healing. Big or small, life's events and traumas are stored in the tissues, nervous system, and brain, and they don't forget without healing intervention. Like archeologists, we're looking for the holy grail, and we'll find it within by cleaning and clearing the inner obstacles. Unless we go beyond the muscles, the joint problems remain unresolved, and the trauma will follow us wherever we go.

Avita is a revolutionary approach to pain, not because we manage it but because we get to the source of it. We learn to work *with* the symptoms instead of alleviating them. It can be a challenging shift in thinking, but the sooner we catch the symptom and follow it to the source, the better off we are. And that's Avita at its best because we use the shapes to find the issues before they find us. Avita can detect the restrictions deep in the joints and surrounding fascia the same way a massage therapist discovers and releases tight tissues. Once you experience the benefits and learn a little about your body's healing physiology, you may be inspired to find and resolve all of your restrictions.

As we touched on earlier, Avita can be helpful at any age but can seem like a waste of time for a young, fit body because it does not foster a sense of exhilaration and achievement. I sometimes say if you are not attracted to Avita Yoga, it's because you are either not old enough or you haven't had chronic injuries. I am reminded of a beloved student who discovered Avita at eighty-three. John always had sage, often humorous advice. He wished he had found Avita Yoga at seventy-nine and described aging as a slow-motion injury. Thank you, John.

THE DISORGANIZED BODY

You can start practicing any time but keep learning. The better we understand the things that work against us, the more equipped we are to maintain a practice for lasting health and mobility. The general idea is to shift from a *disorganized* body to an *organized* body.

In simplistic terms, we could say that a disorganized body is out of alignment or has "bad posture." Yes, people feel better after having bodywork to release tension and help body parts "stack up" with better structural alignment. However, the reorganizing process happens at a level deeper than the structural components of muscles, bones, and connective tissues. The best reorganization happens when we include the nervous system and our separating thoughts, beliefs, feelings, and memories that lurk in the unhealed mind. Want the best results for any yoga or bodywork? Let the work reach you at levels beyond the physical.

In a disorganized body, the neuromuscular-skeletal matrix is fragmented and inefficient. It's like a computer that hasn't rebooted in years. As unhealthy as it is, we unconsciously habituate to it and make it our reality, our temple. We rationalize the pains, adapt to them, and accept them as part of our identity. As the body, brain, and nervous system adapt to disorganization, we get comfortable with the discomfort. When this happens, we resist doing anything that challenges the body and mind to organize and feel better. The ego resents change and will find illogical excuses not to practice or move in a new and healing direction.

Organized or not, we adapt to the current homeostatic state. The body and mind do their best to hold it all together and do what you ask. Whether it be lying on the couch, working at your desk, or pedaling on your bicycle, everything on the inside of your body continually adjusts to deliver what you ask of it on the outside.

In classes at the Ida Rolf Institute, we were taught to evaluate bodies and spot the disorganization. It's easy to assume that an organized body with "good posture" equals a happy, pain-free life. But we know that's not always the case. It is better to ask, "What does disorganization *feel* like?" If something doesn't feel right, let us welcome it and work with it. Rolfers and other bodyworkers are trained to see the disorganization—Avita shapes are designed to help you *feel* and simultaneously resolve it.

Remember, we use the shapes to resolve conflict in the body *and* the mind. It could be nervous energy—fear, anxiety, guilt, loneliness, or a need to stay busy. It could be feelings of lack and uncertainty carried in the background of your mind everywhere you go. How much effort and strain does it take to be happy and content? None. Our yoga is to get underneath the presenting conditions and symptoms and bring the core issues to the surface where they can be resolved. In Avita we use physical disorder and discomfort as a means to heal on all levels, and while the shapes give us countless clues and gentle guidance, we don't assess the body from an outer-alignment perspective.

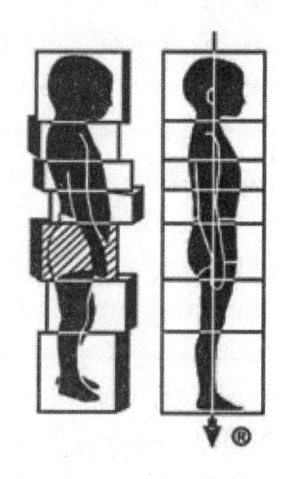

The Rolfing logo depicts a disorganized (left) and organized structure (right).
Image used with permission of the Dr. Ida Rolf Institute

Suppression is the conscious inhibition of unacceptable impulses, memories, feelings, or desires. Repression is unconscious inhibition of the same, and both occur because of our fear of facing them. The healing process involves allowing grievances and upsets into awareness, where we can feel them, express them, and let them go. The yoga is gentle and poignant. By welcoming the impulses, memories, and feelings, instead of inhibiting them, we can identify and release them. It's a timeless formula that works.

Said another way, freeing ourselves from *samskaras*, the limiting mental impressions from the past, liberates the mind and helps us experience positive changes in body and in life. It is essential to create a space where we can practice safely without fear of judgment or friction, as this allows us to become more in touch with our limitations and address them effectively. Metaphorically speaking, we "upgrade" the software along *with* the hardware. We use the time in the shapes to resolve the physical restrictions and blockages while unwinding the nervous system and creating healthier neurological pathways. For lasting results, they must both be addressed.

If our yoga is to find and bring the problems to light, there will likely be some unpleasantries along the way, like spasms, cramps, and other annoying-but-healing sensations. Spend a little time in the awkward shapes and watch how quickly you and your body reorganize around the newfound information. In a sense, we work backward through time to unwind the body and mind. In this way, the body and mind can work hand in hand to generate health and happiness. It's a beautiful thing.

The reorganization starts to feel so good that, at some point, we *want* to find the limiting restrictions, beliefs, and values. We take the yoga off the mat and into our lives, where life itself shows us the judgments and thoughts that keep us in fear and uphold a sense of separation. Be kind and patient with yourself. The smallest *willingness* to go within is the only requirement for meaningful change. If the Avita practice is for you, you will know it because you will feel it. Be vigilant for any desire to advance the shape alone, for outer accomplishment can be a decoy for the inner work.

You don't have to alter your lifestyle or behaviors; just plant the seed for a better way. Let it seep into your bones, and helpful reorganization will come. I've seen it work even for ardent nonbelievers. We don't seek change; we let the changes come *through*. Some students tell me that they weaned themselves off medications while others started feeling better and forgot to take them! Many have found solace and health through Avita, never dreaming they would be "doing yoga." Linda, one of our yoga students in her mid-seventies, mentioned in a Christmas card that she is practicing yoga. I can only imagine the comments she received from friends and family. Avita is for everybody. Practice, and all else will follow.

THE ORGANIZED BODY

The organized body is like a well-maintained vehicle. Alignment may not be perfect, but there is little to no pain, no restrictions to practical movement, and no compensation patterns. It moves freely and recovers from stressors quickly.

In the truest sense, the organized body is a reflection of the liberated mind. As we release stored physical and emotional baggage, we develop a distaste for its accumulation. The mind becomes clear and calm. It's not easily alarmed and is far less susceptible to cravings, mood swings, and emotions. When the mind is at rest, the body, regardless of its condition, becomes a reflection of the healed Self.

CHAPTER 3

It's All About the Feedback

When we practice, the eyes are usually closed, allowing the mind to draw inward, where we slip into the role of the peaceful observer. We don't have to think or evaluate. The cues are verbal and thorough. If you practice with me online, you may glance at the screen occasionally, as a student in the classroom might glance at a neighbor to ensure they have the right idea, but then your attention returns to the inner feedback, the sensation.

Is it too much or too little?

How do you know if it's safe and helpful?

This is the yoga. Discernment for healing sensation is the primary skill you will develop and improve upon. It is a skill you *can* perfect, and it's entirely different than trying to perfect the shape itself.

LET'S PRACTICE

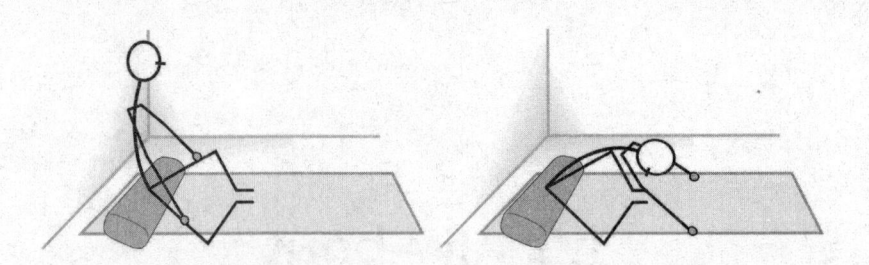

Sit on a bolster or firm cushion with your back supported against the wall and your tailbone a palm's width away. Place the soles of your feet together with heels about twelve to fifteen inches from your pubic bone and relax for about thirty seconds to let your body and mind adjust to any feedback. Without using momentum or a sudden movement, draw your abs in and slowly come off the wall with the intent to flex your lower back. You may use your arms and hands by gripping your knees to help. Let your head soften forward, and relax the upper back, shoulders, and rib cage. To do it any other way compensates for lower back rigidity. The aim is to encourage the entire spine to curve forward. Feel into your hips and move according to the feedback. Stay in this position for one to two minutes and rise if the sensation becomes too intense. Can you be discerning for the healing sensation? Can you avoid evaluating the position and *be* with the yoga? Reverse the process and draw the belly button toward the wall behind you to come slowly back up.

Scan the QR code to access Let's Practice video:

This inner listening and guidance that come with the shape are priceless. It includes the nervous system as it fosters freedom, health, and peace of mind. How would the results last if we didn't bring the nervous system along for the ride? If we override this critical feedback, we negate the reparative process by pulling past conditioning into the present moment—and we end up getting in our own way.

For over two thousand years, yoga has been about the mind and our ability to get out of our way to allow healing to come through. This remains true, so watch your thoughts. Watch the relationship you build with the sensation and the shape. Watch for the deterrents to real progress: judgment, evaluation, and doubt. Do you want to heal? Do you want to feel better? Would you like more peace and ease in your life? Then *listen*. Refrain from overriding the feedback. Stop telling the old story—to yourself and others. Is there a willingness to relinquish control, loosen the grip, and allow something different to come through? At some point, we must stop the repetition that brings the same undesirable results. Look within and find your healing power. Miracles happen when we listen, wait, and judge not. It's time to expect miracles.

IMMEDIATE FEEDBACK

Immediate feedback comes with the shape moment by moment. Most of the time, it should feel like welcome and sustainable pressure in and around the joints. If there is degeneration or arthritis, it will feel scratchy, irritated, and sometimes a bit abrasive, but it's welcome. If the feedback is deep organic pain especially around the hips or shoulders you must reduce pressure. It can also feel stretchy at times, but it's not a stretch. We "stretch" only enough to encourage a muscle to release, soften, and become more supple. We never attempt to stretch to make muscle tissue longer.

In essence, immediate feedback is the barometer to help you gauge the proper degree of effort, depth, or pressure. Avita shapes have passive and active components, and because passive shapes can bring strong feedback, we never force relaxation in any shape. Sometimes a shape is held, supported, or adjusted until the tissues reorganize and the nervous system is ready to let go and relax. In this way, many "earn" their way into passive shapes by actively holding them until the day comes when they become passive and relaxed. You will hear these details during practice. Instead of seeking comfort in the shape, we kindly find the restriction and disorganization, which is why Avita teachers never give cues like "Just do what feels good to you." It misses the entire point of practice.

We do not eliminate sensation, nor do we go looking for it. Too often, students protect the problem by supporting the shape, but again, *we cannot protect our way to better health*. The shape must be sustainable without eliminating sensation, and we use immediate feedback to stay in or adjust the position.

Sometimes the immediate sensation is strong because of the steady activation of the muscles. It can border on pain, and you are working too hard if you clench your teeth, tighten your face, or feel the need to breathe through your mouth. In these situations, please reduce pressure or leave the position to regain a peaceful sense of self. The effects of practice will keep working for hours after you stop, so there's never a need to push. Do what you can and come back another day when you will often feel the results of your work.

Avita is a potent practice, so you must keep your mind observant, continuously determining what is truly helpful and what is not. This reflective listening with heart and mind is the meditative part of the practice.

Sometimes the experience of being in a given shape will be relaxing, and sometimes not. It will depend on your history, constitution, recent activities, demands, emotions, diet, and so on. Many factors dictate the information one receives during a class. That's beautiful because multiple benefits can come from embracing one sensation, and we don't need to define the results. We just feel better. Befriend the feedback, make it sustainable, and helpful changes will come with minimal effort. Let's not adjust or manipulate our bodies or lives because we are *supposed* to. Let us practice and walk through life *listening* for intuitive guidance.

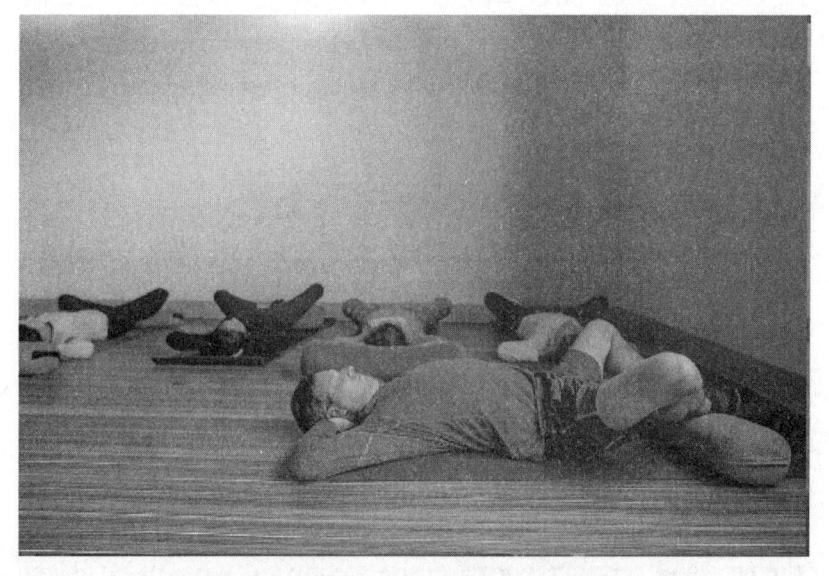

The feedback will change with time and practice, and so will you. It's essential to tune in, not out. The shape will improve if and when it's supposed to.

We are not all wired the same way. A shape that is intense to one person may provide little feedback to another. Sometimes you may relax in a shape with little to no sensation. It's okay. You're still benefitting from the time and pressure. Pushing for sensation is risky. Increased sensation is *not* the goal and can lead to injury. Remember, peace is our primary desire because it's the only consistent guiding reference we have in life. Peace always brings the most favorable outcome. With experience, you may settle into a shape with strong feedback or sensation and be okay with it because you are confident, certain, and peaceful.

In other words, don't skip steps! It's essential to simultaneously unwind the nerves, fascia, mind, muscles, joints, and bones. Shortcutting comes with a cost. If we skip steps, they will need to be repeated at some point if you want the result. Patience is a characteristic of a good student, and patience is a state of mind: confident and sure of the outcome. Remember, we are reorganizing the body and mind for optimal health. The pursuit of fitness is an entirely different goal. In Avita, we don't override the curative moment—we thrive on it.

DELAYED FEEDBACK

Sometimes feedback comes later, up to twenty-four hours after your practice. Please pay attention to it but refrain from evaluating it and jumping to conclusions. Many will feel diminished pain and improved mobility after their first class. They walk better. People often experience a sense of relief because it is the first time in years they have come close enough to the problem to address it. For some, once the pain is gone, they decide to stop practicing. However, most students will continue with a desire to unwind more patterns and restrictions, which means that informative, sometimes uncomfortable sensations may arise along the way.

Are you willing to work with feedback that touches on the pain as a means to get closer to the problem—where it can be solved? This question is as valid for the body as it is for the mind in day-to-day life.

Delayed feedback from an Avita class can come in the form of a dramatic loss of energy that sometimes borders on exhaustion. It's not because we're working "hard." It's because we are working *deep*. Remember, the shapes are potent because they access the fascial network interwoven *everywhere* throughout your body. An immeasurable number of proprioceptors are located in the connective tissue, meaning we cannot reorganize the hardware (the bones, joints, and muscles) without involving the software (the nervous system and brain).[7]

For some, the early stages of an Avita practice are a little like recovering from surgery. I have had students drop out of practice because of exhaustion that set in a few hours after class. It's an unproductive feeling, but if they had continued a little longer, their systems would have reorganized, and they would have crossed this threshold, found increased energy, and realized how productive practice can be.

Welcome the feedback. In the early stages, you, too, may feel an energy drop after practice later in the day. It's normal. If you can, take a nap. It's your body and mind in healing mode. If it's unbearable and downtime is impossible, pace yourself. Doing only the first half of a class is okay in the beginning stages. Two classes per week are enough for some. Find your healing rhythm and pace yourself in the short term for long-term results. As your body reorganizes, you will experience an increase in stamina and energy. You might even develop the ability to nap during practice. It's a sign that we *need* the rest. Snoring is occasionally heard in the classroom, and we consider it an indication that the yoga is working perfectly—and it gets a few heartfelt chuckles from those nearby.

Remember the primary goal of the practice? *Peace.* It's important here because, while sensation is the barometer that indicates the degree of pressure you apply to your body, peace is your primary goal and guide. If the sensation is strong enough to "take your peace away," reduce pressure and regain your peaceful center. That said, it's remarkable how much intensity a body part can channel in a healing direction if you are truly confident *and* calm.

Sometimes the sensation can be almost unbearable, but you decide to stay with it because you are certain it is helpful and not harmful. But again, don't push it. When in doubt, reduce pressure. It's far better to come back another day. Get to know your thresholds and pace yourself.

The final point about delayed feedback is the importance of bringing it to your next class. Bring your pain and work *with* it. Talk to your teacher about it. Pain is information, and you will learn to use it wisely in Avita classes. Bring your worries, bring your concerns, bring your stress and stiffness, bring your "stuff" to practice. Avita is *for* these things, not to hide or diminish them. We often call upon a positive attitude to make it through difficulties, but that can avoid the deeper work and delay healing. It's not honest. Positivity can become a form of self-deception if it pushes helpful but uncomfortable information down that wants to come up for resolution. It's a delay tactic that maintains separation when feelings of insecurity are covered by false confidence. In Avita, we don't fake it till we make it. The fantasy of a positive attitude overlooks the problems and keeps them lurking below the surface where they remain hidden and problematic, exactly where the ego likes them. If you *want* peace and health, be honest with yourself and those around you, and let the obstacles to confidence come up. It's our yoga.

MUSCLE CRAMPS—FRIEND OR FOE?

Most of us know the agonizing sensation of a muscle cramp. Often painful and frightening, spasms or cramps are sudden, involuntary muscle contractions. I think of them as a neurological response that occurs when joints and muscles move into new territory.

In Avita, like other sensations, muscle spasms and cramps are not to be avoided. They arise when we use muscles more thoroughly to investigate new joint movement. Can you see how perceiving cramps as dangerous and avoiding them limits potential? If you search the term online you will find information on treatment and prevention, but to prevent cramps and think them harmful is misguided. If we avoid cramps, we protect the problem and maintain a limited range of motion. It goes back to the myth discussed earlier of protecting the problem through pain avoidance.

Muscles, bones, joints, and connective tissues work in concert with the nervous system and brain to maintain your current state of health and range of motion. Avita Yoga is meant to interrupt, unwind, and reorganize the parts and systems that may be unpleasant at times. Practice will build new and improved relationships between *all* the moving parts. Healthy adaptations occur as you break free of old patterns and let the muscles react and reorganize while steadily moving into new territory.

To be clear, I'm not talking about muscle cramps that could be related to nutrition or hydration. Yet even well-nourished and hydrated practitioners experience muscle spasms and cramps from shapes that move them into a greater range of motion.

So, what causes a cramp? Is it in the brain? In the joint? A triggered memory? Who cares! We don't need to know. A new and unfamiliar nanometer of movement is enough to set off a chain of events that upset the often comfortable degree of movement. If we avoid the cramps and spasms, we succumb to the dysfunctional patterns behind them. Cramps will come and go until we learn to ride them out and use them to clean up the underlying conditions that cause them.

Think of cramps like unexpected guests at your door. Turning them away would be reactive and unkind. At the same time, we wouldn't "make a scene" and rush in to hug them. We "dance with cramps" by welcoming them to unwind their cause and make the muscle supple again. We need not be afraid of these uninvited guests. While uncomfortable, unwinding cramps does not have to be painful if we welcome them and work with them.

DON'T SHOOT THE MESSENGER

Pain is not the problem. It's a signal that informs us that something inside needs our attention. Without it, we'd have no way of knowing that something isn't quite right. If we're willing to listen, the pain will lead us to the source of the problem, where it can be resolved.

You've heard the axiom "Don't shoot the messenger." It's sage advice to avoid being upset at someone delivering "bad" news. The messenger merely provides the information and is *not* the source of the problem. The ever-impatient ego cannot see past the judgment to the truth. Assigning cause to the messenger and killing it in a futile attempt to alleviate the torment of the message breaks communication and leaves us without helpful information.

The messenger and its message have value. When we seek only to lessen or kill the pain, we shoot the messenger when it could provide helpful information. Pain not only leads us to the problem but also monitors our progress along the way and lets us know if we are on track. As we unwind problems at their source, life opens up in miraculous ways that no shortcut could ever make possible.

If we can't eliminate the pain, often we try to numb or deaden it with food, alcohol, drugs, or distracting behaviors—anything to avoid honestly looking directly at the problem. Why? Because numbing preserves a problem that is upholding a desperate, separate, and seemingly "safe" sense of self. It keeps the ego in charge and furthers its cause to keep us afraid, disempowered, and alone.

Instead of doing the inner work, we avoid unpleasant thoughts and feelings that drive them deeper. We kick the can down the road, but eventually, we realize we want to go beyond symptom alleviation and look directly at the problem. This is when real healing begins because fear begins to fade away.

Our ability to *eliminate* pain advances continually. The medical industry revolves around pain and has many ways to "make the pain go away," but the underlying cause often remains. Be careful not to give your healing power away. Get the outer help and relief when necessary, but don't let it deter you from the reward of doing the inner work. It's tempting to go for the quick fix, but if we must eventually work through and not around the darkness to get to the light, is an instant remedy really more direct and time-saving?

Powered by the mind, Avita Yoga relies on the body's healing physiology to solve the problems at their source. Once you shoot the messenger, it's gone. Armed with another option, perhaps we won't be so quick on the draw.

HEALING SENSATION

Have you ever seen cows or horses lying in a pasture? Sometimes they lay on their side, but often they rest with hooves and legs curled under and their bodyweight on their hips, knees, and ankles. The pressure on their bones and joints is proportionate and appropriate for each animal. Would they do it if it didn't feel good? The pressure must feel inherently beneficial and nurturing for a cow to stay in the shape and chew their cud, which they only do when relaxed.

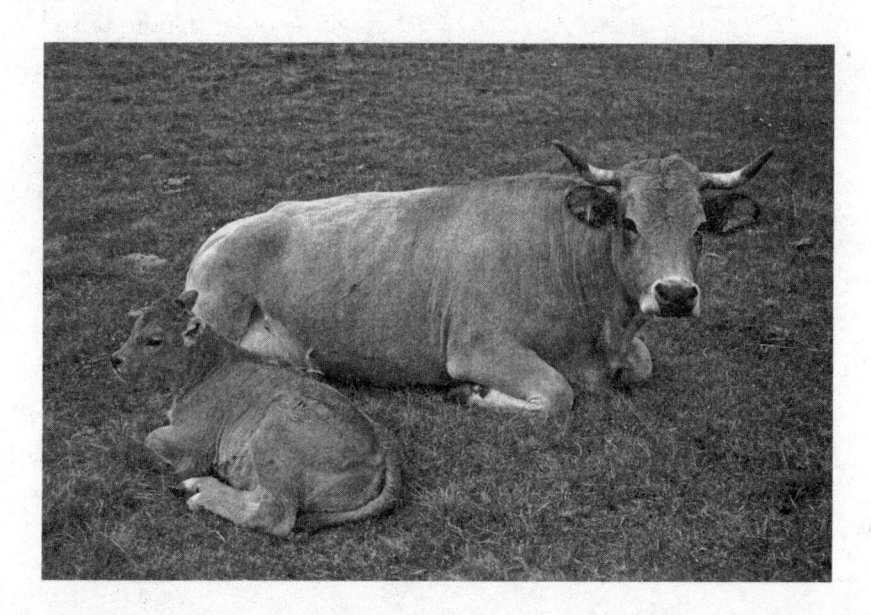

Quadrupeds lie like this for long periods before making subtle shifts to a different shape. Watch your pets. They do the same thing. Why? I say it's because they enjoy the meditative quality of healing sensation. It's natural. Look closely, and you can see it in their eyes.

--- LET'S PRACTICE ---

Kick off your shoes, remove your socks, and sit toward the edge of a chair. Bend one knee and rest the top side of your foot and toenails on the floor. Fold up a blanket or towel to add some cushion for your toes if needed. Sit back, relax, close your eyes, and observe the position while letting the feedback come to you. There's nothing fancy about it, but can you feel the release in the ankle and instep of your foot? Can you feel the flexion on your knee? Stay here for about thirty seconds, then slowly slide the foot forward, adding more compression and sensation to your big toe. Don't make it painful. Make it sustainable. Can you be here for another minute or so? When you release, don't stretch or eliminate sensation. Shift to the other side of your chair and repeat on your other foot and toe. The shape targets the big toe, but for those with a lot of knee rigidity, it's also a safe and effective entry point to begin generating flexion on the knee.

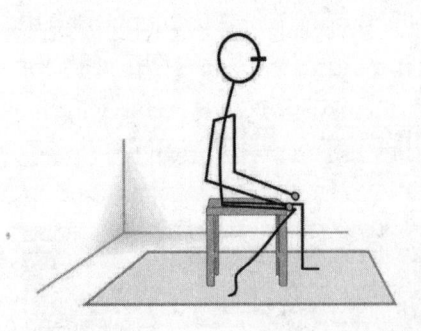

Scan the QR code to access Let's Practice video:

BONES LOVE PRESSURE

Because we are so conditioned to protect and avoid unpleasant sensations in and around the joints, let's do a quick review. Earlier we discussed the impossibility of protecting or preserving our way into better health. When we protect, we weaken and impair full functionality—regardless of the body part. If we don't use a muscle or joint to its potential, we gradually lose it, and more often than not, the pain signal can be years in coming.

Sometimes, under a doctor's advice, we use weight-bearing activity to stimulate bone density. We know that bones and joints don't do well without gravitational impact. On the other hand, too much, too fast can be injurious. Steady, nurturing forces are different; they are healing, meditative, and deeply calming to the mind. The sure way to injury is to skip steps in the process and move too fast. Instead, slow down and get to know your body and its potential, regardless of your age. Avita aims to kindly go through and not around the restriction.

At first, the pressure from the shape is hard to trust and understand because we've learned to avoid it. Contemporary wisdom says, "If it hurts, even a little, avoid it." This is where Avita shines. There is pain that harms and discomfort that heals. With practice, you soon get a feel for the healthy difference and continually refine your practice over time.

The healing feeling may sometimes be intense but still nurturing and inviting. Something inside says, *Okay, you can trust this.* Reduce pressure if it takes your peace away or doesn't feel welcome. Breathing too hard? Ease up. Yogic alignment comes not when body parts are lined up but when the mind is peaceful, relaxed, and joined.

The practiced Avita student knows what *healing sensation* is and understands how unique it feels in various body parts. The nervous system picks up the sensory input from muscles, tendons, joints, and the surrounding connective tissue and brings the information to your awareness. We spend time in the shapes and tap into the healing sensation by adjusting the pressure according to the moment-by-moment feedback it provides.

In class, I often suggest, "Find the sensation that invites you in. Too much too fast is not sustainable." A student once asked me how she would know if it was too much pressure. I said the sensation would be disturbing and take your peace away. She said, "Oh like fingers on a chalkboard?" I replied yes. If you don't know what a chalkboard is, imagine screeching in your earbuds. It's grating. You wiggle, squirm, and can't wait till it's over. And because students often look around the room and compare themselves to others, they quickly grow impatient and try to reposition themselves into what someone else is doing. They don't realize that a sixty-five-year-old woman further into the shape has been practicing for a year or two and has resolved many obstacles.

Further does not equal better. How far we advance in form has no bearing on the benefits of *being* in the shape, in the healing power of *now*, *with* the relevant feedback. Healing sensation can have a bittersweet quality that is mesmerizing. As fulfilling as it may be, it has a limit. When in doubt, diminish pressure or come out and wait for the next shape.

If you advance the shape too quickly, time won't be on your side, and tension will get pushed to other body parts to support the painful area, which will uphold the compensatory patterns we are trying to resolve. For example, the neck and shoulders may tighten because the sensation is too intense in the knee. The idea is to dissolve restrictions and dismantle the holding patterns that foster pain and limitation. It is a skill that you will naturally develop, and it will serve you on your yoga mat and in your daily life.

Start slowly. Treat fear or doubt like a restriction and work with it until it resolves. In short, leave nothing out. Allow all thoughts, feelings, and memories to surface along the way. It's part of the healing journey. Take time to learn the difference between "pain" that heals and pain that harms. It might be intense for a moment, and then it dawns and you say to yourself, *Wow. Yoga is not as scary as I thought. It's not what I'm accustomed to, but I could spend some time here.* These are potent and powerful moments. Students walk away from class with a whole new mindset, feeling better than they had in years. Why? Because they befriended "the enemy" and gained some freedom. The class and the time in the shapes were enough to begin cleaning up the problem. The yoga is cleansing as much as it is mobilizing.

Want practical insights into the healing power of compression? Watch the movie *Temple Grandin*. It is a true story about the courage to be oneself. Born with autism, Temple did not fit into the world in a conventional way. As part of her healing journey, she used compression to relax her body, calm her mind, and transform her liability into a gift to herself and the world. Like Temple's "yoga," our yoga must be practical on every level. Temple's single-minded approach to life is an inspirational example of following love's intuition against all odds. She has inspired me in countless ways.

Part of the Avita teacher's job is to help students understand the difference between pain that pushes you out and healing sensation that lets you in. The former takes your peace away; the latter brings it. Demanding too much from your body in the shape can unnecessarily increase your heart and breath rate. Thoughtfully and kindly, we meet and greet the feedback, which slows us down and drops us into a peaceful presence necessary for healing.

Students with specific or chronic issues must experiment with the boundary of movement and explore the pain. Sometimes the feedback gets a little gray or uncertain because we initially interpret unpleasant sensations as pain to be avoided. Go slow and remember: You may not like the feeling, but your joints love it.

Healing sensation can be felt universally throughout the body. While one part may be targeted and have stronger feedback, it does not detract from your ability to observe your entire body from a place of peace. That's true whether we are active or passive in the shape. For example, can you feel the work in your hands and fingers while observing the relaxed nature of your feet and toes? You know you're safe when you can be active and engaged in one part of the body while simultaneously observing the rest so that no one part steals the show. With practice, we start to realize the holistic nature of the mind, and we learn to leave nothing out. Can you feel your mind everywhere in your body at once? It's our yoga to have an all-inclusive approach, which reflects the universal nature of the one love we share.

LET'S PRACTICE

Take a break and lie on your back with your knees bent and your feet on the floor. Support your head, close your eyes, and bring the right knee toward the right shoulder. Interlock your fingers behind the thigh and let gravity initiate the movement. Slowly apply pressure so that there's a nurturing compression in the fold of your hip and groin. Any stretchy sensation in the back of the thigh should match the compressive feeling in the front of the hip or groin. You control the degree of pressure to find healing sensation, and a peaceful state of mind. When in doubt, reduce pressure, especially if there is deep organic pain in the groin. This can be indicative of a torn labrum and should not be pushed. If the feeling is peaceful, maintain the shape for one and a half to two minutes. Release the foot to the floor and repeat on the left side.

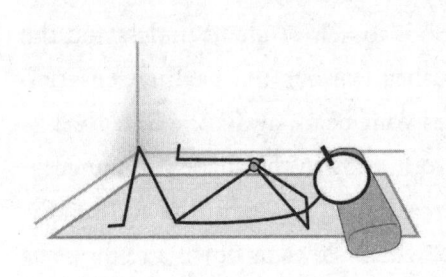

Scan the QR code to access Let's Practice video:

THE SENSATION OF TIGHTNESS

Muscles are not tight of their own doing. They are under the constant influence of the brain and nervous system. They are innervated, meaning the nervous system governs the movement, relaxation, looseness, and tightness of muscles. If we turn the nervous system "off," which happens under a general anesthetic, a tight muscle becomes a flaccid muscle. So, if we pursue a tight muscle and try to "stretch it out," we unwittingly miss the source of the problem.

Unfortunately, we often avoid the sensation of tightness and move around it to continue using the body the way we want. Consciously or not, the *brain* picks up on stiffness and finds the most efficient way to move around it. The *nervous system* adjusts quickly and constantly in the background to keep you doing your desired activities. As part of a "survival mode," the *body* will make endless compensations for the rigidity so that you can keep moving. It's part of the programming that says, "Oh, there's a stiff area. Let's avoid that and focus on the parts that move freely. Let's make this little adjustment and keep the body moving." This continuously occurring, internal process contributes to the aging process and limits our lives.

We are programmed to take the simple path, which becomes the road well-traveled. Avita takes the road *less* traveled. Finding the avoided places and parts makes all the difference. As rigid areas start moving again, circulation increases, health improves, and lost movement is found. To achieve these results, restricted areas must be located and welcomed into our practice. Instead of advancing the shape and slipping into the compensation patterning described above, we slow down and welcome the stiffness. Why? Because if you feel it, it means you found it, and your yoga is working on it. We sometimes see students bypass blockage or restriction in the classroom because they want to move quickly to attain the "desired position." We often say, as teachers, "You get points for going slow," because we know good things happen when we slow down for the "speed bumps."

People on the tighter end of the spectrum get the feedback instantly. If anything, they would love *not* to feel their bodies so much. They despise the discomfort of stretching and tend to avoid yoga, dance, and anything that requires the demonstration of flexibility. Isn't that good feedback? Yes. Let it be helpful and approach your yoga practice accordingly. Those who say "I can't do yoga because I'm not flexible" are the very ones that Avita serves well. Amazing things happen when we stop trying to stretch and instead drop into shapes that reach the bones and joints and unwind the restricted fascia around them. Fascia morphs; muscles do not.

THE SENSATION OF NO SENSATION

On the other hand, people with flexible constitutions get very little feedback, so they go looking for it. These individuals love feeling "the stretch" and want more of it. They tend to push themselves in yoga, dance, ballet, and gymnastics. In a constant quest to feel the body, it's easy for these people to disorganize themselves, which leads to imbalances in their structural matrix. In a sense, flexibility *is* the problem because their joints and bones are not carrying their proper share of the load, which means the muscles often feel tight. And so, they feel the need to stretch because it feels so good. But there's a risk in stretching muscles in a body with a flexible constitution. It can destabilize the structure and lead to problems down the road in the form of degeneration and arthritis. More than anything, their bones and joints need compression to foster stability, not more flexibility.

Almost everyone has a joint or region that does not produce much sensation under pressure. Still, we do not seek for more sensation. It's the wrong goal.

THE SENSATION OF WEAKNESS

The prescribed answer to weakness is usually a strengthening program. But if you look closely at the sensation of weakness, it is often a by-product of pain and restriction. Pain can short-circuit healthy muscle innervation and leave us feeling weak and imbalanced, as discussed earlier. As we go through our day, we unconsciously move around the limitation and pain, which exacerbates the problem. Whether in the body or the world, compensation patterns are born when we avoid the issue. We don't want to look at the problem because it will slow us down, albeit temporarily.

Consider that a slight limp from knee pain can become a lifelong hobble if left unchecked. A limp, like using crutches, is meant to be temporary. With a thoughtful therapeutic approach, we can target the problem with proper shapes, move *through* the limp, and return to a natural gait.

If a significant amount of time has passed since the pattern began, the student will find themselves moving into a shape with lots of quivering, shaking, and spasming of the muscles. Most would rather avoid this "embarrassing" feedback, take control, and accomplish the shape. But I'm always encouraging Avita students to be patient and spend time in those areas of perceived weakness and uncertainty. Those are golden moments where reintegration and reorganization occur. It is far more beneficial to get to know and work with the sensation of weakness instead of trying to overcome it and gain strength. Remedy the problem, and the healthy "wiring" is restored.

This weakness I'm referring to usually goes unnoticed in the gym during fitness training or weight lifting, because the goal of strengthening alone and building muscle definition overrides the less integrated areas. The muscles that can handle higher demand become more robust, while the smaller, unused muscles and the nerves that supply them get left behind and buried in a weight-lifting regimen. Lifting weights or strength training is okay, and I would never advise against something you enjoy. Many have successfully supplemented their favorite activities and fitness programs with Avita. Yet in my experience, weight training alone is a poor substitute for the more profound work of *undoing* the barriers to strength. Muscle strengthening is very different from maintaining bone and joint health and resolving the fascial restrictions.

"Over and over again, people come to me, and they tell me, You just don't know how strong I am. They say "strength" and I want to hear "balance." The strength idea has effort in it; this is not what I'm looking for. Strength that has effort in it is not what you need; you need the strength that is the result of ease."
—Ida P. Rolf, Ph.D.

Hidden problems eventually surface, so why not save time and catch them early? Be very clear about the desired outcome of your physical routines. Practice all-inclusive shapes and movements to find the sensation of weakness and condition your joints, bones, and muscles together. Muscle tone occurs naturally in Avita because we use all three elements thoroughly and because of improved circulation as restrictions resolve. Our immune function improves as we enhance the movement of lymph. Digestive problems resolve as we restore lower back flexion and exert compressive forces on the abdomen.

In short, you want more than strong muscles alone.

FEEDBACK—FROM THE MAT TO LIFE

Can you comprehend the difference yet between practicing according to the feedback vs. pushing for an outer goal? When we override or overlook the insight from feedback, it's often because we seek to attain an outer image of what we perceive as good and healthy. Listening is a crucial and practical part of our practice because it leads to intuitive guidance. It's how we learn to get out of our way and take the road less traveled. Unimaginable good begins to happen as we let go of our limiting beliefs. In Avita Yoga, we use the body, the shapes, and the inquiry because it takes us through fear and anxiety to the love and serenity on the other side.

When you learn the difference between pain and healing sensation in the shapes, you can naturally transfer that training to your entire life. That is the crux of this book—the critical takeaway. As we learn to accept the body's feedback without judgment, we can learn to accept life's feedback without judgment. Are circumstances disturbing? Do you want something in your life to change? Do you feel anxious, stressed, or pushed? Who's pushing? What seems to be taking your peace away? It's *all* feedback. Listen to it. These are the obstacles to peace. You have the power to dismantle them, for nothing outside your mind can take your peace away without your permission. Learn to differentiate healing sensation from pain, and you will soon learn to discern the difference between love's intuitive guidance and the ego's fearful reactions in all you do.

*"Change your thoughts, and
you change your world."*
—Norman Vincent Peale

DON'T ELIMINATE THE SENSATION

After sustaining a shape, we naturally want to "shake it out" or do something to eliminate the residual sensation. It's habitual and often subconscious. The underlying thinking is that this feeling I'm having is bad, and I need to do something about it. In Avita, we take the opposite approach and view the elimination of residual sensation as an interruption to the healing process. We let the body figure it out. We don't shake anything out. Instead, we may rest and observe or go directly into another shape that changes or uses the work from the previous shape to get results through another. We don't interrupt the stimulation that inspires the inner healing physiology.

It works in day-to-day life as well. Shaking a mental funk is like erasing a physical sensation from an Avita shape during practice. Instead of getting rid of it, try observing the funk. Befriend it. See if you can watch it without judgment. Emotions are the feedback of some underlying thought or belief. Instead of glossing over them, follow them in so you can get to the bottom of the underlying condition where it can be dissolved once and for all.

For example, you may believe that *all* people should yield to you when entering the highway from an on ramp. The belief sets you up for the thought of being a victim. The thought of being a victim sets you up for the emotion of anger. Change your belief and happiness will follow. The cost of upset is enormous. This is the yoga of getting to the underlying conditions that keep us stuck.

CHAPTER 4

Our Trepidation with Joints

The ego's pain-avoidance programming also comes with the idea that we must protect our joints. As mentioned, we cannot preserve our way into health. That's why Avita Yoga goes deep. It targets the body's deepest structures: bones, tendons, ligaments, and the joints they construct. If you are accustomed to working with the superficial nature of muscles, it may take courage to slow down and resonate with sensations you thought to avoid until now. Develop a consistent practice, and you'll be thrilled with the results. Take your time, and don't override the feedback. With Avita Yoga, you can stay healthy and mobile for a lifetime. Muscles have stolen the show far too long. It's time to start caring for our bones and joints. First, let's zoom in on the interplay between joints and several closely related functions.

LIGAMENTS, TENDONS, MUSCLES, AND BONES

Being informed so that you understand the parts and how they work together is beneficial, especially when discussing with a therapist or doctor.

We like to think of the body as a collection of parts. Anatomists "draw the line" and break it into subsets of systems, tissues, and cells, yet it's all perfectly seamless. Tendons merge with bone, which connects seamlessly with capsule linings and ligaments. And while it's nearly impossible to discern the starting and stopping between a muscle, a tendon, and a bone, it's helpful to play along and consider the anatomy of ligaments, muscles, tendons, and bones, and the components of structural support and movement.

Ligaments are fibrous bands of tissue that connect bones. They are made of collagen, a vital protein that provides flexibility and strength, helps stabilize joints, and prevents them from moving too far or too fast.[8] **Muscles**, which are made of muscle fibers, contract or relax when stimulated by nerves to produce movement.[9] **Tendons** are tough tissue bands that form a seamless transition between bone and muscle. Primarily containing collagen, both tendons and ligaments provide resiliency and strength.[10] **Bones** are the rigid structures that make up the skeleton. They provide support and protection for the body's organs. Bones are made of calcium, phosphorus, and other minerals.[11]

Ligaments, muscles, and bones work together to create movement and support for the human body. In summary, ligaments connect bones to bones, tendons join muscles to bones, and the contractions of muscles produce movement.

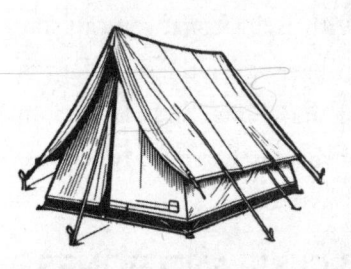

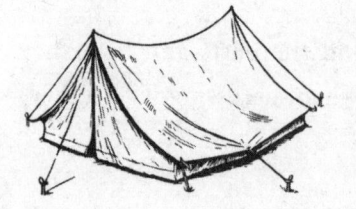

This is a helpful analogy I learned in Rolfing school and not to be taken literally. Consider the way a camping tent holds its shape. The poles are analogous to our bones. The lines or ropes that support the tent are the tendons and muscles. The tent fabric is like fascia that holds everything together.

If you tug on any one part, everything moves. Ideally, the components are well-balanced and interdependent. Together, they create a multidimensional form that can move and adapt to its surroundings.

If the tent is too rigid, it can't adjust to a strong wind—and damage may occur. Too much flexibility causes the tent to lose stability and integrity. Our bodies are not much different.

Here are some specific examples of how ligaments, muscles, and bones work together:

- When you bend your arm, the biceps muscle contracts, and the elbow flexes.
- When you walk, the muscles in your legs contract and relax to move your legs.
- When you jump, the ligaments in your knees help stabilize the joint and prevent it from buckling or overextending.

Ligaments, muscles, and bones are all essential for movement and support. In a perfect environment, they work in concert, but when any of these structures is compromised, it can affect the function of the others. For example, a torn ligament can make it challenging to move a joint, and a muscle strain can cause pain and weakness in a joint. But we are getting a bit granular. Let's not focus on the superficial nature of muscles and acute injury. We want to explore the bigger picture and the impact of time, pressure, and gravity on the components we rely on for support and movement.

SYNOVIAL JOINTS—THE TARGET

The human body has about 360 synovial joints, mainly in the limbs, that allow for a wide range of movement and are essential for practical activities such as walking, running, and lifting. We target synovial joints in Avita Yoga, and for maximal health and mobility, we aim to access them *all* through an ongoing progression of sequences.

The six main types of synovial joints[12] are:

- **Ball-and-socket joints:** Examples include the shoulder and hip joints. They allow for a wide range of movement, including flexion, extension, abduction, adduction, rotation, and circumduction. Their enormous potential range of movement, coupled with our tendency to lose it over time, makes these joints prone to arthritis and degeneration.
- **Hinge joints:** Examples include the elbow and knee joints. These joints allow movement in one plane, such as flexion and extension. Both are prone to arthritis due to uneven use, which contributes to the degradation of overused parts and the resorption of underused parts. These joints are also subject to sports injuries and imbalances from quick lateral and repetitive movements.
- **Pivot joints:** Examples include the atlantoaxial joint between the first and second cervical vertebrae, which allows the head to rotate; and the joints between the radius and ulna, which allow the hand to pronate and supinate. These joints offer rotation around a single axis. Because pivot joints are used in habitually small ways with minimal mechanical load, they can lose cartilage and bone density sometimes beginning in our twenties and thirties.
- **Condyloid joints:** Examples include the wrist and knuckles. These joints allow movement in two planes, such as flexion, extension, adduction, abduction, and circumduction. They are found at the base of each finger, but not the thumb; at the base of each toe; and in the ankles and wrists. Condyloid joints are easy targets for overuse and underuse, making them prone to arthritis.
- **Saddle joints:** Examples include the carpometacarpal (CMC) joint of the thumb, the sternoclavicular (SCM)

joint of the thorax, and the calcaneocuboid joint of the heel. These joints allow for movement in two planes, similar to condyloid joints, but with more freedom of movement. The base of the thumb is a saddle joint, and like the others, when imbalanced, it becomes a common area for arthritis and pain.

- **Plane joints:** Examples include the joints between the metacarpal bones of the hand and those between the cuneiform bones of the foot. These joints allow for gliding movement and can become arthritic when disoriented.

GRAVITY, PRESSURE, AND THE LACK THEREOF

We must look beyond fitness paradigms to find a lasting remedy for joint pain, arthritis, and degeneration. Diet, exercise, and movement alone are not enough to solve joint issues.

Now that we have identified the structural components, let's look at the unique impacts of gravity (or lack thereof) and practically apply what we have learned to everyday life on Earth. When astronauts spend time in space, the absence of gravitational force negatively affects their bodies. Most notable is the loss of muscle and bone mass. In the absence of gravitational force, muscles weaken and atrophy and bones lose structural integrity and density, similar to the conditions of osteoporosis. It can take up to 70 days for an astronaut to walk normally after returning from space.[13] Incidentally, until they invent a gravity machine, I sometimes think Avita Yoga could be a way to stay healthy in space.

What can we learn from this? It's the universally recognized principle in action: Use it or lose it. If a lack of gravity or pressure negatively impacts muscles, bones, and joints, can we systematically apply pressure to them to increase bone and muscle health? Yes, and there's scientific physiology to support this. But first, a word about trust.

It's very helpful to understand the science and physiology beneath your skin that keeps bones and joints healthy, but our yoga cannot rely on science alone. As you read and practice, consider the essential characteristic of *trust*, which I'll define as our ability to rely on something we cannot see. We can't see what's happening inside the body, but we trust that taking a vitamin or eating certain foods will result in the desired outcome. We have all learned to trust things and processes we cannot see. Heartfelt intuition, our best guide to life, remains hidden if we don't *trust* and follow it.

I've noticed that results come quicker and last longer for those with a natural propensity to trust the Avita practice. They "leave doubt at the door." Of course, true trust is not blind. We could say that presence, trust, and intuition are the same because they all lead to miraculous experiences.

Like heartfelt intuition, the healing physiology that cleanses and remodels joints and bones constantly operates in the background. It's our yoga to find, nurture, and rely on it. Can you develop trust in that? This is where the physical and spiritual practices of yoga are beautifully intertwined.

BONES AND JOINTS CAN BE REMODELED

By understanding the physiological characteristics of osteoblasts and osteoclasts, we can better understand the remodeling process and how it contributes to bone and joint health. Hormones and nutrition play a role, but perhaps most impactful on bone health is *how* we use our bones and apply pressure to them. Bone remodeling is a continuous process that involves removing old bone and forming new bone to maintain bone strength and structure.[14]

Osteoblasts are responsible for *forming* new bone. They are derived from mesenchymal stem cells and secrete proteins that form the extracellular matrix of bone. These proteins include collagen, osteocalcin, and alkaline phosphatase. I remember osteoblasts' name and function because they "blast bone into place," but in fact they accumulate and transform into osteocytes or bone cells where pressure is induced. Pressure is also the driving force for unwanted bone formation, as in the case of bunions and tori that result from clenching.[15]

Osteoclasts are responsible for *resorbing* old or unhealthy bone. Remember the video game Pac-Man? Like that round, yellow dot-chomper, osteoclasts are multinucleated cells that attach to bone surfaces and secrete acids and enzymes that break down the bone matrix. They show up where there is damage and disease, but they also show up where there is a lack of use or pressure.[16] Isn't that interesting? The body is designed to dissolve and remove that which is not being used. It's practical. The body won't tolerate anything that is idle. If it can't be resorbed and eliminated, it will calcify, store, or restrict it. Nothing in the body happens by accident.

The activity of osteoblasts and osteoclasts is tightly regulated to maintain the crucial balance between bone formation and bone resorption. When the balance is disturbed, conditions such as arthritis (bone or joint inflammation), osteoporosis (bone softening), or osteopetrosis (bone hardening) can develop.[17] Osteocytes are equipped to detect external stress loads and thus manage the remodeling process.[18]

Osteoblasts and osteoclasts communicate through various mechanisms, including direct cell-to-cell contact, cytokines, and extracellular matrix proteins. Changing hormones, activities, and the impact of gravity and pressure tend to alter this communication. When this intimate balance is disrupted, bone and joint problems can develop. But there's one more key ingredient to the healthy balance of any joint: synovial fluid, which I affectionately refer to as "elbow grease."

SYNOVIAL FLUID: JOINT LUBRICANT

Synovial fluid is clear, viscous, and found within our joints. It is produced by the synovial membrane, a thin layer of tissue that encapsulates the joint. Synovial fluid has several vital functions, including:

- Lubrication: Synovial fluid helps to lubricate the joint, reducing friction and allowing the bones to move smoothly.
- Nutrition: Synovial fluid provides nutrients to cartilage, the tissue that covers the ends of the bones in a joint.
- Shock absorption: Synovial fluid absorbs shock, which helps protect the joint from injury.
- Immune function: Synovial fluid contains white blood cells that help to fight infection.[19]

The main components of synovial fluid are:

- Hyaluronic acid: A glycosaminoglycan that gives synovial fluid its viscosity. It helps to keep the fluid thick and slippery, allowing the bones to move smoothly.
- Lubricin: A glycoprotein that coats the surface of the cartilage. It helps to reduce friction between cartilage and bones.
- Proteins: Synovial fluid contains various proteins, including enzymes, antibodies, and growth factors. These proteins help speed the healing process and neutralize harmful substances in the joint to keep it healthy.[20]

Just like the components of bone and cartilage, synovial fluid is constantly being produced and resorbed. The rate of production and resorption is balanced to maintain the correct and healthy amount of fluid in the joint.

Can you see the importance of keeping synovial fluid healthy and clean? What would happen to the tissues it bathes if the fluid became toxic or unhealthy? Would you bathe in the same dirty water day after day? Of course not. Your body naturally cleans and replenishes the synovial fluid within your joints, but it depends on movement and pressure, two things we shy away from as we age. Avita Yoga is a way to regain and maintain youthful movement.

METABOLISM, ENERGY, AND WASTE BY-PRODUCTS

Every metabolic process in the body uses energy to create new building blocks—each cell contains its own energy-producing power plant. And anytime energy is produced, toxic by-products are made. The body utilizes a complex process of circulation and elimination to move toxins out of the cells and tissues through solids, fluids, and gases, and eventually to the outside world. The body is like a factory with various customized manufacturing rooms. Each room has its specialty and uses raw materials to create energy, building blocks, and waste. If toxins accumulate inside the building, the environment degrades, and the workers get sick. It's the same in the body. Within each synovial joint, cartilage and bone undergo constant metabolic change and thus generate toxic by-products, which are released into the synovial fluid. If the fluid is not cleansed and renewed, it becomes "dirty bathwater" and, in time, can lead to degeneration. Even in a perfectly healthy body, the toxic by-products of cartilage and bone remodeling must be handled, or fluid clarity and function will be compromised.[21] Would you ask for better working conditions if you worked in a dingy, unkempt factory?

Blood and lymph pass through tiny, one-cell-thick vessels and capillaries. However, small vessels like this would get crushed inside a joint, so nature placed them in the synovial subintima. How is fluid cleansed and renewed within a synovial joint? The short answer is *pressure*. Kind, consistent pressure is cleansing whether it is active or passive. When you make a strong fist, muscle contraction's force on your knuckles pushes the fluid through the cell membrane into the intercellular matrix outside the joint. Try it and observe your fingers and the sensation. Can you hold it for two minutes? When you release, can you rest into the sensation and avoid "shaking it out?" Observe and try not to interrupt the healing physiology that's taking place. With practice, you will become aware of the kneejerk reactions to sensations and feelings that you determine to be "bad" and the unconscious need to "fix" or interrupt it.

Synovial joints are aptly named for the membrane that encapsulates and retains the synovial fluid within. The outer part of this membrane is called the synovial subintima and contains the microscopic vasculature where macrophages and white blood cells help remove waste products from the fluid inside the joint cavity.

This cleansing process is called microcirculation.[22] The capillaries in the synovial membrane are one cell thick, which allows for the exchange of nutrients and waste between the vasculature and lymphatics. But how does this occur? The action of compressing and releasing the joint *is* the pump. The system relies on movement and pressure differential in and around the joint.

The lymphatic vessels around the joint capsule transport the fluid to lymph nodes and the spleen, where it is cleansed before being dumped back into the bloodstream. Unlike the vascular system, the lymphatic system has no pump; it relies on movement and pressure differentials to move it in the right direction. Otherwise, it becomes stagnant, which results in swelling and inflammation.[23]

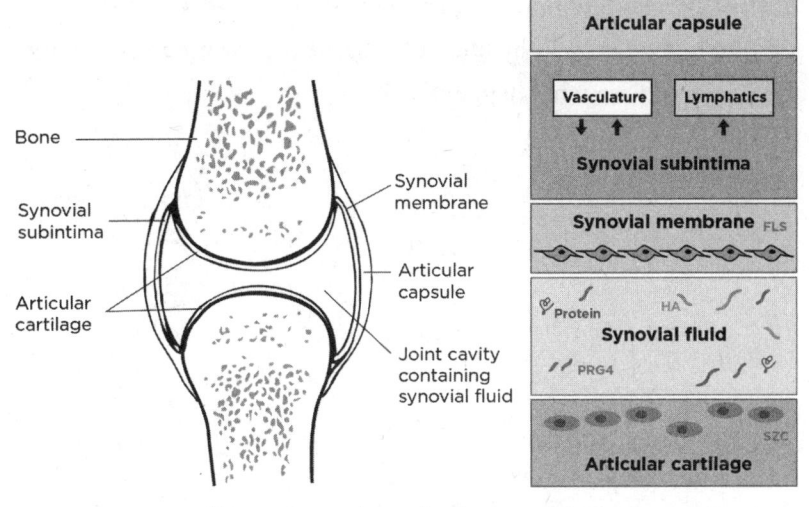

These two illustrations show the layers of tissues and the movement of fluids from deep articular cartilage to the more superficial vasculature. Articular cartilage attaches to bone. The joint cavity contains synovial fluid and this is contained by the synovial membrane. The vasculature and lymphatics are enmeshed in an intracellular matrix that form the synovial subintima. The outermost layer, known as the articular capsule, is comprised of fascia.

In Avita Yoga, we target the lymphatic system as much as anything else to get the fluids moving, which promotes health and boosts immunity. It's one reason we do so much work at the wall. Unlike headstands and handstands, Legs Up the Wall is a doable shape for most people and can be sustained long enough to get results.

Age, injury, infection, and various diseases can impact our ability to cleanse and restore the joints, but let us be slow to blame and quick to take gentle responsibility for our health and state of mind. The composition of synovial fluid alters during an individual's lifetime due to changes in mechanical loading and joint degeneration. But which comes first over a lifetime? The lack of adequate use and pressure, or slow-motion degeneration? It doesn't really matter—the solution is the same. Why not add consistent pressure to your bones and joints and see what happens?

The playful activities of youth keep the joints healthy, but as time passes, we tend to blame the past for our health and joint problems today. These limiting thoughts and beliefs are not helpful. Take gentle responsibility and begin anew.

ARTHRITIS

Now it's time to talk about arthritis, a term used to describe a joint disorder. When researching the term, you'll find a list of symptoms and remedies, but you'll have to look deep for a descriptive cause. Consequently, we often perceive and treat arthritis as an ailment independent of potential causes, like the food we consume and how we use or don't use our joints. Unless we slow down and examine our lives, problems like arthritis and bone degeneration become more of a mystery than they actually are. It's why we wind up treating the symptom rather than the problem.

Let's take the mystery out of arthritis. For any lasting solution, we must get close to the source of the problem where it can be corrected. When we do this, amazing things start to happen. We could even call it the *miracle mindset*.

While the degenerative result is similar, there are two kinds of arthritis we will address: rheumatoid arthritis (RA) and osteoarthritis (OA).[24]

Rheumatoid arthritis is an autoimmune disease that causes inflammation of the joints. Autoimmunity is when the body's immune system mistakenly attacks healthy tissues, including joint lining, which can lead to pain, stiffness, swelling, and damage. RA can affect any joint in the body, but it most commonly strikes the hands, feet, wrists, knees, and elbows. The joints become brittle in RA due to pannus, an abnormal layer of fibrovascular tissue that degenerates the joints. Treatment typically involves biologics to decrease the inflammation and destruction of the joint, but gentle exercise is also often recommended. Avita Yoga can be very helpful with the symptoms. Applying kind, sustained compression with a slow release can help ease the pain, but because RA is a systemic issue, it can also be fruitful for these folks to look deeper into other dietary or lifestyle themes to get closer to the cause and find helpful remedies.

If you search for the cause of osteoarthritis, you will find these usual suspects: wear and tear of joint cartilage, age, obesity, genetics, and joint injuries.[25] When we have difficulty getting to the root cause of an ailment, we tend to name it as a disorder or disease. While terminology is always debatable, "arthritis" seems to have been upgraded to degenerative joint disease or DJD.[26] All my life, I have found it beneficial to look beyond the labels.

In my experience, the list of causes mentioned above is not consistent enough to be given that much damaging power. For me, osteoarthritis occurs when toxins accumulate in the synovial fluid, causing the cartilage that cushions the bones to deteriorate. Cartilage may wear away, but it can also "resorb away" if not used adequately. We are quick to find blame and slow to ask probing questions. It's not always a matter of overuse or repetitive movements that lead to the loss of cartilage.

According to the Mayo Clinic, "The most common type of arthritis, osteoarthritis, involves wear-and-tear damage to a joint's cartilage—the hard, slick coating on the ends of bones where they form a joint. Cartilage cushions the ends of the bones and allows nearly frictionless joint motion, but enough damage can result in bone grinding directly on bone, which causes pain and restricted movement. This wear and tear can occur over many years, or it can be hastened by a joint injury or infection."[27] Along with most sources, it suggests "wear and tear" as the problem. Saying that wear and tear is the cause of arthritis is like saying rain causes flood damage. Is it rain causing the damage or is it mismanagement of the structures that direct the flow of water? I'm taking a strong position on this, and it's my experience that we need to redirect our attention to adding pressure to joints. I hope others will pick it up and do the research.

Others will suggest poor diet and unhealthy lifestyle choices are contributing factors. Yes, but we must look for a more profound common denominator to this widespread pain that is costing time and money to millions every day.

Poor diet, smoking, and wear and tear may be contributing to arthritis because they all add to a toxic buildup inside the joint capsule that inhibits remodeling and healthy metabolic processes. I'm all about addressing these things, and there is an excellent book, *Healthy Joints for Life* by orthopedic surgeon Richard Diana. I appreciate the title. Dr. Diana goes into incredible detail on the science of arthritis, nutrition, and helpful exercises. But what if there was a way to cleanse the joint and promote healing and mobility? What if the solution was staring us in the face?

OSTEOARTHRITIS

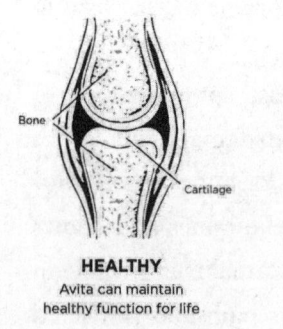

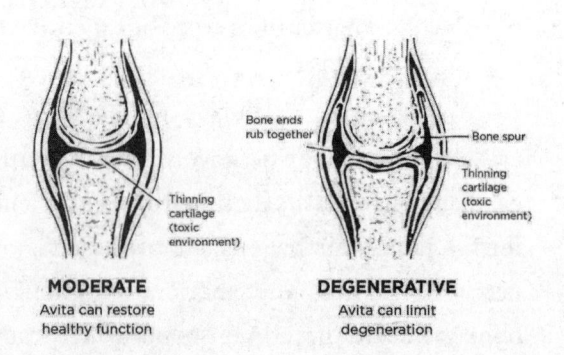

HEALTHY
Avita can maintain healthy function for life

MODERATE
Avita can restore healthy function

DEGENERATIVE
Avita can limit degeneration

What if the buildup of toxins in joints creates a degenerative environment that inhibits the remodeling process and leads to joint pain, stiffness, and swelling? Osteoarthritis most commonly affects weight-bearing joints, such as the knees, hips, and spine, but not because they bear weight. From an Avita perspective, it's from a lack of full, passive, and active use and the cleansing pressure it generates. I have found that compensation patterns resulting in asymmetrical contact on the articulating joint surface are a contributor. This, combined with the fear and avoidance of working with the pain and introducing thoughtful cleansing and compression, leads many down the road to weakness, degeneration, and ultimately sometimes a diagnosis of osteoarthritis.

The good news? You can address both osteoarthritis (OA) and rheumatoid arthritis (RA) by applying compress and release forces on the bones and joints. Genetics, aging, and lifestyle are the usual and often innocent suspects. But again, rather than find blame, it's far more helpful to take gentle responsibility, which always includes a healthy dose of forgiveness that brings us into the healing power of now, where helpful insights and corrective action occur.

While Avita can help manage the painful symptoms of rheumatoid arthritis, it can bring remarkable results to osteoarthritis patients. Why? Because it unwinds compensation patterns and remodels the joint's interior. We use the shapes to find imbalances and apply mending pressure, which stimulates the healing characteristics of the underlying physiology. As always, the sooner we catch it, the better.

Disclaimer: If you have pain or swelling in a joint, it is essential to see a doctor to get a diagnosis and treatment. Treatment for synovial fluid conditions may include medication, physical therapy, or surgery. A rheumatologist can use lab results to help determine the type of arthritis you have.

FIBROMYALGIA

Fibromyalgia is a long-term health condition that leads to pain and tenderness throughout the body. More common in women, symptoms include muscle pain, brain fog, fatigue, face and jaw pain, digestive problems, and insomnia.[28]

There's no definitive test for fibromyalgia, and diagnosing it is often part of a differential diagnosis—a medical process of elimination. Fibromyalgia is a dynamic condition, which means people won't experience symptoms in any specific order. There's no road map to know when and how fibromyalgia symptoms might affect someone.

Rheumatology nurse and Avita Yoga teacher Andrea L. Lawrance, RN, suggests "maintaining your overall health can help reduce the severity of fibromyalgia symptoms." She has found that Avita Yoga, as a relaxation technique to reduce stress, is most helpful to those with fibromyalgia. "Reducing stress is vital to the body and its underlying tissues and systems. The yoga activates a parasympathetic response to slow the heart rate, lower blood pressure, increase blood flow to muscles, improve digestion and sleep, diminish fatigue and anxiety, improve concentration and mood, and reduce pain."

People with conditions like arthritis, depression, anxiety, emotional trauma, or severe injuries are more likely to develop fibromyalgia.[29] Andrea reminds us that "fibromyalgia can have a significant impact on one's life, but many with fibromyalgia experience fewer flare-ups with mild symptoms when they exercise regularly and moderately and include calming yoga practices like Avita to harmonize the mind." She acknowledges that through movement, we find health.[30]

OTHER FACTORS AFFECTING JOINT HEALTH AND MOBILITY

We are each born with joint variations, but how we walk through life, and repeatedly move or don't move, affects joint-surface health and range of motion. Joint health is a function of its *total* use and movement. For example, a hip joint may be able to move back and forth, such as when walking or jogging, but if it loses its ability to rotate externally, its health will be compromised. All joints become less healthy but not necessarily painful as full movement potential is lost. As we have discussed, the discomfort that leads to joint replacement usually comes later, and later could be tomorrow, which is why I encourage consistent practice *now* to maintain joint health for life.

Think about it. The body pushes problems down and buries them to keep us going, but nothing gets repressed forever. One day, you may bend over to pick up a ball, and your back "goes out," or your hip starts hurting. It is far better to start today and bring the issues to the surface so you can resolve them. Why not adopt a simple maintenance program, the same way we schedule and maintain the health of our motor vehicles?

I hope you are beginning to understand that range of motion and movement quality affect the health of our bones and joints. Still, two other unsuspecting factors impede joint health: muscle and fat. Too much of either can "insulate" and limit healthy joint compression and movement.

If fat accumulates or muscle bulks in the movement space, then joint mobility is compromised. We don't need space in the joints; we need it *between* body parts for movement to occur. Too much belly fat inhibits our ability to curve the lower back forward into its full range of motion. Likewise, too much muscle around the shoulders impedes the ability to reach fully overhead. And so on. Excessive fat or muscle inhibits movement, which may only become problematic when articulating surfaces degrade as adequate joint compression is lost. It's an example of how extremes work against us.

"Too much muscle" might sound counterintuitive, but I've met bodybuilders with rock-hard abs and severe degenerative issues in the lower back. The mindset is to keep strengthening. They continue doing what they've always done because it holds the pain at bay. But for how long? Beware of the *muscle trap*. More of anything can quickly get the best of us.

Whether you experience fat accumulation or muscle bulking, please let it be the helpful motivation to start down a simple path devoid of extremes. As you go, be vigilant for thoughts of blame and guilt—they keep us locked in the past where the solution is not available.

CHAPTER 5

Protocol for Joint Replacement

I've seen the results of many joint replacements, and most of the time, students are happy with the outcome . . . but not always. I've observed all kinds of unsuspected complications. As advanced as the technology is, most prefer to keep the joints they were born with.

Jump into an Avita practice sooner rather than later, and you will increase the probability of maintaining, if not growing, the mobility, health, and freedom you have today. With consistent practice focusing on particularly troubling areas, you can clean up arthritis and degeneration and maintain your original parts for life. I call that a home run. But let's look deeper for those rounding second base with an irritated hip or knee.

COMPENSATORY PATTERNS AND JOINT REPLACEMENTS

As life happens, we bump against the body's limits and the accumulation of knocks, bruises, pains, breaks, and strains. At some point, we become weary of the pain and want a quick fix. There is a proper time and need for joint replacement, but let's not put the cart before the horse. For proper function, we have to look at the cart *and* the horse.

While we can replace a worn and degenerated joint, we cannot replace the patterns that brought the problem on in the first place. You may swap out the joint, but the pattern *behind* the problem remains. This pattern and our way of moving will affect other nearby joints and bones because the replaced joint is exceptionally robust compared to nature's softer tissues. Fabricated from plastic and metal, it has no nerve endings for feedback, so the patterns are required to move *around* the body's new, most stable and secure part. The movement pattern that caused the need for replacement gets pushed elsewhere in the body, which can add strain or stress to other structures and supporting tissues.

How do compensation patterns work? If you've ever tried to walk with one big toe that doesn't move well, you already know. If the big toe is calcified and won't bend, compensation patterns will get pushed throughout your body. The same goes for walking with one knee, hip, or shoulder that isn't working optimally. You feel the changes in your gait.

Unless compensatory patterns are addressed, the replaced joint can push the pattern that started the problem in the first place to the next weak link in the system. Similarly, if the postoperative range of motion is left incomplete, it can add to the underlying movement pattern.

Artificial joint replacement or not, we need a way to resolve the compensatory patterns that bring the problems on. Modern medicine can replace many physical parts, but it cannot replace the software that governs the nuances of movement. Can you see how the puzzle pieces all fit together? The software of the nervous system interacts with muscles and fascia to create grooves in the bones, and in turn, the deformations of the joints feed the patterns in the muscles, tissues, and brain. Compensation patterns work perfectly against us.

> *Healing pressure can remodel the bones and joints, but the Avita approach simultaneously reorganizes the connective tissues and the nervous system, where debilitating patterns are enabled.*

Doctors seldom root out the criteria contributing to the damage because they are trained to target and fix the presenting problem, not the behaviors and patterns that lead to it. We may be surprised at the diagnosis, but we're quick to assume age, time, and overuse are to blame. Yet there's more to it. What about that weak ankle or that stiff knee? Could it have contributed to the movement pattern causing the need for hip replacement?

I remember a student who started coming to class because of shoulder pain about a year after a replacement. It took us about a month to realize that the surgical implant was moving inside the humerus. The implant portion was slipping when it should have been stable. She went back for a second surgery, and after PT, we worked steadily to identify and unwind the patterns in her neck, upper back, and chest. These patterns had placed excessive pressure on the original joint and, thus, on the shoulder replacement. Shoulder patterns are complex, and shoulder surgery rarely results in a full range of motion. For this and other joint replacements or repairs, it's essential to understand and respect the anticipated post-surgical range of motion. Keep in mind that habitual compensation patterns and restrictions in the soft tissue may limit the potential range of motion of your new joint. Learn these things from your doctor and develop a good working relationship with your PT. Ask questions.

I know others who had a succession of joint replacements before they knew about Avita Yoga—one knee, one hip, the other knee, and the other hip. Can you see the importance of identifying the pattern behind the problem? We don't have to decipher or intellectualize any of it—we need only practice the shapes that reveal the patterns and unwind them.

DECISION-MAKING—TO REPLACE OR NOT

Let's be honest: Big or small, decision points can push us into a fearful place where we feel isolated and alone. I have found that once a person is informed about the degenerated joint in question and a replacement is recommended, the decision to proceed is often cast in stone. We cannot tolerate the "bad news" and the detailed information about the ugly problem that's going on inside. It's scary and painful, and so we want it out. Now! Spontaneous decisions can be heartfelt, but it's wise to let time be on your side and use it to watch your mind. Do the research, do the yoga, and with a healthy dose of humility, let it empower you to make a heartfelt decision. Still unsure? It might mean you have more time. Delay is okay. It gives you time to include others in your decision-making process, so the ultimate choice comes with a joyful feeling.

Surgeons are taught to collect the data, isolate, and repair the problem. It's what they do best, and we can be grateful for it. It's up to you to take a broader perspective. Just because we are under a doctor's care and become patients does not mean we should stop being patient students. Keep using your Avita practice to inform you. I know it's not easy, but try not to let the pain push you into a rash decision. Remember, pain is a messenger. Only *you* can broaden the scope to consider the things that will bring the best results, which often includes garnering the help and insights of others.

Keep in mind also that artificial materials behave differently than bone. While you might be ready to resolve the pain and get on with your life, the feedback from that part of your body will be different going forward. It's considered good news to most, but it isn't reassuring for some. I know this from speaking to students who describe *the feeling of no feeling* where the replacement occurred.

People tend to research the doctor rather than their own movement patterns and restrictions. This book is meant to help you do the inner work for a better outcome whether you opt for surgery or not. Learn about your body parts ahead of time. Find out what your current range of motion is. It's measured in degrees, and you should know what it is before surgery and the expected post-recovery range. A physical therapist can help with this; why not choose one *before* your surgery and make an appointment to get their insights? They can evaluate your condition, measure your current range of motion, and provide advice. They've seen it all, both before and after surgery.

Interview the doctors. Ask questions and learn about the replacement parts and the surgery itself. Many undergo surgery and are surprised by their discoveries, thoughts, and feelings afterward. Get involved and give your procedure the same attention as when shopping for a house or a new car. We rarely buy the first car we test drive. It's okay to get a second and third opinion. Dr. A might have been excellent for your friend's procedure, but would Dr. E be a better fit for yours?

Is the recommended replacement joint designed for a full range of motion? If not, why? Post-surgery, you'll keep working to achieve full range. In many cases, the longer you wait, the harder it will be to recover because scar tissue will form to support the limited movement.

Ask more questions. Why is replacement model X being recommended for you? The doctor may use only one brand or model, but find out why. Ask about the incision(s). Where and how big? Are there options? What muscles and tissues will be cut or impaired during surgery? What are the chances of nerve damage? Are there movements you should avoid post-surgery? How do people with your body type, age, and lifestyle fare with this particular surgery?

PREHAB BEFORE REHAB

So, let's say you've made a thoughtfully considered decision to replace the joint. What next? What might you do to best prepare for surgery? Ideally, you've delayed the surgery and been practicing Avita three to four times a week for three to six months. If your class does not have the specific shapes for your problematic joint, you are doing your daily "homework" to target it. You're on it. This pre-surgical approach can feel aggressive, but you remain kind and consistent with shapes that target the problematic joint. This dedication will prepare you for surgery and might allow you to avoid it altogether. You can learn about "homework shapes" in the online workshops at avitayogaonline.com/featured-workshops.

If you have decided to replace the problematic joint, read on for the pre-surgical Avita protocol, which can be particularly helpful. Is there a risk in experimenting a bit? Knowing the replacement is probable, why not use the time before surgery to prepare? Some surgeons have a pre-surgical protocol that is similar to the one I've seen work for Avita students. They want patients to start up to six months in advance. The prehab involves strengthening exercises that challenge the joint's range of motion to prepare the surrounding soft tissues for the replacement. Avita prehab is similar but focuses less on strengthening and more directly on the joint, the surrounding connective tissue and the nervous system. It's less work and more targeted, and it will teach you that working with the pain to find a healing sensation is okay. More on this later.

Prior to surgery I recommend three to four weekly Avita classes to promote mobility and resolve compensatory patterns as soon as possible. Problematic joints need the focus, but never at the expense of avoiding the full spectrum of classes. Dissolving restrictions in the ankles and hips, for example, means a knee replacement will be received and integrated more readily. The entire body needs attention to promote the best mending and integration of any one body part. Why? Because no part is apart from the whole.

Once you have decided to replace the joint, we go deep. Six to four weeks before surgery, I recommend going into the pain and fear with two or three key shapes every day and holding the shape for one to two minutes. It may be intense initially, but the pain should diminish as time passes. You know about feedback now, and you are listening to it. For helpful guidance, you can find thirty-minute sessions online that target the major joints, including the feet, knees, hips, hands, and shoulders. Once on the website, you can filter the classes by session length and search for the body part you want to address.

Why this depth and focus? Why do I suggest going *in to* the pain and fear? Because that is necessary to release and remodel the fascia around the joint that has organized itself according to the limited joint movement. The joint will be replaced, but the surrounding tissues will not. There's no better time than *before* surgery to undo the programming that accommodates the pain and limited movement.

In addition, while this protocol will help prepare you for surgery and the intensity of the PT afterward, it may also bring results that change your mind about the procedure. Please share this information with your doctor and physical therapist, welcome their feedback, and listen to their advice. Watch the tendency to get wrapped up in the timeline and the doctor's schedule. It's not too late to change course. Do your prehab and consider staying on schedule even if openings come sooner. Good decisions are never based on guilt or fear.

Stop your physical practice and rest three days before surgery to reduce any irritation or inflammation. You are ready, and your recovery will be quicker. You've set the tone for post-surgical rehab and a sustainable practice that will keep the parts moving well.

We do the prehab to instill the healing aspects of Avita into the bones, joints, and soft tissues and reprogram the nervous system. It plants the seed for the important PT and continued yoga and self-care that will follow. This is hard to conceive, but those with years of Avita practice are less accident-prone, and if they do have an accident, they recover faster. From vehicle collisions and skiing accidents to falling down stairs, many have shared stories with me of how astonished they are at the speed of their recovery because they had the yoga in their body and mind before the accident. If an injury occurs, practiced students know how to work with pain and use the shapes to facilitate the healing process.

On a final note, the medical technology for surgery and joint replacement is impressive and ever-improving. You can replace a joint and be home the same day, but it will take time and determination to unwind the underlying patterns in the surrounding tissues and nervous system. If you anticipate surgical replacement, consider this protocol before and after surgery:

1. Beforehand, use Avita shapes to work on the tissues in and around the joint. Do this three to six months before the anticipated surgery date and practice three to four times per week. Find the recommended shapes in the featured online workshops and hold them for one to two minutes.
2. After surgery, do your physical therapy. Near the end of the PT, use the same recommended Avita shapes to gain a full range of motion and integrate your new joint.
3. Consistent practice will help you accept and integrate your newly replaced joint. Use Avita to resolve patterns, reorganize the body, and redistribute the workload.

CHAPTER 6
The Spine

The spine moves by spreading small amounts of motion across many vertebral bones and joints. If movement in one small part of the spine is restricted, then the rest of the spine must compensate for it. Blockages in the spine sometimes occur where vertebral joints are fused—naturally or surgically. Once part of the spine is fused, the adjacent vertebral joints take on the added burden because where there were two or more moving bones, now there is one. The adjacent non-fused joints carry the extra demand that was previously more dispersed.

When practicing Avita, understanding and respecting the transfer of movement to adjacent joints after one or more are fused can help keep all the adjacent bones and joints healthy. It's important to maintain the proper movement long after surgery to avoid negatively impacting the nearby joints.

FUSION AND STENOSIS

Natural fusion occurs over time and can be asymptomatic. Degeneration within joint space can lead to calcification, which impedes movement. With decreased movement, calcification advances and can result in stenosis, a narrowing of the foramen, the canal through which the spinal cord passes. While more rare, another possibility for pain is degeneration that results in facet joints with excessive movement. There are various surgical techniques to fuse the vertebrae and stop the movement that causes pain. Whether fusion is surgical or natural, movement is prohibited, and both can alleviate pain but may not prevent future problems. Degenerative disc disease, or DDD, has become such a common diagnosis that it is often said to be a normal sign of aging.[31] Is it a disease? Is it "normal," or is it a sign of how we *don't* move? There is no need to assign blame because it's self-defeating and does no good. Instead, take gentle responsibility and watch the changes come through. Perhaps they are a factor, but scapegoating age and heredity diminishes your healing possibilities and insights.

Things that stop moving in nature can become "frozen" or mineralized in place. Hinges on doors and moving machinery parts can rust and "freeze" if not maintained. Joint calcification is much like earthly calcification. Soft tissues become less pliant, and the tissues in and around joints tend to calcify similarly to mineralization we see in nature. For example, immobile vertebral joints can fuse, and we refer to calcified segments of tendon as "bone spurs."

Generally speaking, in the body, where there's movement, there is health. How long would the stalactites and stalagmites in Carlsbad Caverns in southern New Mexico last if there were small but consistent movements in the earth around them—especially if they were encased in fluid (like water) designed to cleanse and carry the debris away? How much movement does it take to keep calcification and arthritis at bay? Not much, as long as it is steady, focused, and consistent, and the earlier you catch it, the better. The movement we are looking for comes in small but steady increments in the form of thoughtful compression to the restricted or degenerated areas. This is the vanguard of Avita Yoga.

THE "DARK SIDE OF THE MOON"

In classes and workshops, I sometimes refer to the lumbar spine as the dark side of the moon. It's out of our field of vision, and we can't feel the lack of movement in the lower back. It may feel stiff, but we are conditioned to avoid the stiffness. It feels so much better to stretch the parts that move, but when we do, the loose places get looser, and the tight places get tighter.

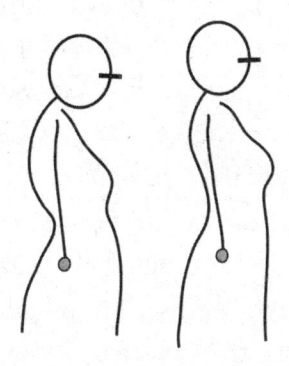

More than likely, the woman on the left has a lumbar spine stuck in lordosis. Mobilizing her lower back is the only way she will, sustainably and without effort, become the woman on the right. To complicate matters, the cervical spine almost always mimics the lumbar spine, so it, too, will have to unwind structurally and functionally.

It took me a while to recognize the pattern. A rigid, lordodic lumbar spine (lower back) often accompanies excessive thoracic flexion or kyphosis (upper back curvature) because it must compensate for the lack of movement in the lower back—and to our detriment, it feels so good and "productive" to stretch and flex the upper back and neck. We've been taught to support the lumbar spine and strengthen the abdominal muscles to stabilize the lower back, but rarely does this bring vital lumbar flexion, which can reduce the chance of stenosis or impede the narrowing of the foramen. Stabilization and support may stifle the pain for a while, but it does not offer the vital movement the vertebral joints need to stay clean, healthy, and mobile.

Well-intentioned yogis who practice the "swan dive" forward fold are trained to "hinge at the hips" and keep the spine straight. It's a graceful movement, and "the forward fold" is elegant, but overstretched hamstrings lose their ability to stabilize the back of the pelvis, and it's very difficult to regain. We'll talk more about this later, but for now, let's drop the rules and appreciate shapes and movements that encourage the multidirectional movements of the spine. When we bend over to pick something up, we don't need to analyze it or turn it into a performance. We want all the coordinated movements of the spine and hips to come together automatically and unconsciously to carry out the task—end of story.

Compensation patterns develop when postural rules are pinned on the body. We should be careful about movement concepts that encourage a particular look or omit natural movement from various body parts. For example, the focus may be on stretching the hamstrings and hinging only from the hip, not the lower back. This is notoriously common in yoga today, where a look is celebrated or a pose achieved.

Warning! If you have lower back pain and/or restriction, do *not* start pushing on your lower back and trying to get it to move. Don't panic, and don't conclude that you have a problem. Instead, we can take a slow and thoughtful approach to introducing movement. A little can be a lot. If you have lower back pain, consider consulting your doctor or PT before beginning a new program like Avita Yoga.

CHAPTER 7

Our Concern for Bones

We know that bones depend on gravity and pressure to maintain health. We also know that bones lose density as we age, starting at about age thirty. This can be especially troublesome for sedentary people or for those who are forced into a passive way of life. Studies have shown that as little as one week of bedridden inactivity can result in substantial bone loss.[32]

OSTEOPOROSIS AND OSTEOPENIA

As we touched on in chapter 4, osteoporosis is the name we give to the loss of bone mass and density over time. Osteopenia is a decreased bone *mineral* density and a less severe diagnosis than osteoporosis. Osteopenia is more typical in women, as hormonal factors are involved. If you go for a bone density test, dual X-ray absorptiometry (DEXA Scan) you'll receive a T score, a mathematical standard deviation that compares your result to the average thirty-year-old.[33] Theoretically, the denser your bones are at the peak age of thirty, the longer it takes to lose it. It's a natural process, and when suspicions arise, we decide to get tested. The results can be scary. I've heard many women fret over their T score. But since worrying our way into better health is impossible, let's look closely to learn more and discover options.

Did you get your bone density checked when you turned thirty? Probably not, and wouldn't it be nice to have that score as a baseline? How would you know your innate tendencies if you obtained your first DEXA Scan at age fifty? The DEXA Scan also targets the thin, outermost cortical layer of bone, where remodeling occurs, but there's much more to bone health and strength than this outer layer. The inner part of the bone may be "spongy" in nature, giving it a resilient quality, but it has a trabecular support system that strengthens and organizes itself along lines of gravitational transmission.[34]

Our chances of taking an unexpected tumble increase as joints degenerate, stiffen, and become painful. The primary concern with osteoporosis is the increased risk of fracturing a bone if one were to fall. But there are many other factors that determine the risk of falling and fracturing a bone. The most significant ones, mobility and balance, are two that we can improve if we focus on them. Think less about strengthening and stretching and more about mobility and balance.

Perhaps the best thing we can do for overall health is to regain and maintain mobility throughout the body. You can find workshops with more details on my website addressing balance and osteoporosis. There's nothing like maintaining a simple, steady practice that fosters mobility, healthy joints, and strong bones. This is where Avita shines.

Like most drugs, osteoporosis medications come with side effects. Some have ramifications if you stop taking them, while others must be discontinued after a specified period. Medications restrain the resorption of bone tissue by inhibiting the function of osteoclasts. Remember the osteoclast? These are the cells that remove bone tissue where it is damaged or perceived as not needed, often due to a lack of consistent joint compression. As we age, everything slows, but there is evidence that healthy osteoblasts depend on fully functioning osteoclasts.[35] They operate hand in hand, and there's a risk of interrupting their working relationship.

What causes bone loss?

- A diet low in calcium contributes to diminished bone density, early bone loss, and an increased risk of fractures.
- Low physical activity diminishes the helpful impact on bones.
- Tobacco and alcohol use decreases the absorption of nutrients like calcium.
- Gender and age play a role; osteoporosis predominantly affects post-menopausal women.
- Race and family history often correlate with diminished bone density.
- Hormone levels can be a factor; lower estrogen levels are linked to osteoporosis.

During middle age, bones lose density and become thinner. With decreased and limited use, the body reabsorbs existing bone cells faster than new bone synthesizes. Osteoblasts cannot keep up with bone-resorbing osteoclasts. So, while the items in the above list are contributing factors, they may not be the cause. As bone loss occurs, the bones lose minerals, mass, and structure, which weakens them and increases their risk of breaking.

We'll all lose bone mass, but we can minimize the consequences. Studies have shown that yoga helps with osteoporosis.[36] Dr. Loren Fishman, MD, has dedicated his life to this topic, with long-term studies using traditional yoga poses to increase bone density.[37] He acknowledges that muscular action has forces greater than gravity. It's how we overcome gravity in day-to-day activities, but more specifically, he doesn't want us to overlook the impact muscles have on bones when we engage them. If this is the case, why waste time building muscle alone, when you can use it deliberately to generate bone and joint health? Muscle tonicity and strength occur as a healthy by-product of using them to target the bones with multidirectional forces that increase bone density.

Unlike yoga styles that focus on stretching, nearly every Avita Yoga shape induces joint mobility and bone strength. Squeezing the muscles against the bone and using them to sustain the shapes has a remarkable benefit to the structural components of your body. Try a few classes and you will feel the difference.

CHAPTER 8

Our Fascination with Muscles

Muscles have a purpose. They use leverage across a joint to move the bones. Large muscle groups comprise smaller muscle bundles made of thousands of muscle fibers or cells. Each muscle fiber, bundle, and group is encased in fascia, creating a vast honeycomb matrix throughout the musculature. Fascia is everywhere. It provides structure, interconnectivity, and integrity. Fascia that seamlessly encases the muscles merges and becomes tendons, which blend into the bone. Anatomical charts show the details and parts, but it's difficult to tell where one kind of tissue begins and ends.[38]

When muscles contract across a joint, bones move. It's how we get around. However, muscles also use leverage and tonicity to support static positions like sitting and standing. In this sense, muscles play a stabilizing role, but it would be too demanding for a muscle fiber to work constantly, so muscle fibers oscillate on and off very quickly to share the load. This is why we "shake" or quiver when sustaining a shape for a prolonged period. This response in Avita shapes indicates inadequate neuromuscular pathways, and working through the shaking is necessary to get results in the bones and joints. In my experience, it's a safe and practical way to reorganize the nervous system. With practice, stamina increases as neural pathways are cleared and renewed. I've seen beneficial results in people with strokes and other nervous system disorders like multiple sclerosis and Parkinson's disease. They appreciate the deep and doable nature of the practice, and while it's not a cure, it can help diminish unpleasant symptoms and reorganize neuromuscular function. Conventional therapy aims at improving function through the refinement of mechanical tasks. In addition, the combination of sustained active and passive Avita Yoga shapes may help regenerate neural pathways in a calm manner that activates the parasympathetic nervous system. Circulation, digestion, and other parasympathetic responses improve, which may indirectly enhance motor function. It's all interconnected.

Again, nothing in the body happens by accident. Muscles don't relax on their own. They have to be instructed to release or loosen. The nervous system and the brain are responsible for a muscle's ability to contract or relax. When one muscle group is activated, the opposing muscles are instructed to relax and extend. This natural contract-and-release response is called *reciprocal inhibition*, and we use it often in Avita to safely release restrictions in the fascial network.[39] Comprehension of simple details like this can be helpful as a yoga student and teacher. Understanding what muscles are and how they work will give us a better idea of how to care for them, and, as you'll soon see, part of our task is to counter many incorrect assumptions about muscles.

WE LOVE THEM

We're fascinated with muscles—their size, appearance, strength, mass, and ability to burn calories. Fitness trends are all about muscles, and conventional "wisdom" says more is better. We love muscles and their look. Popular fitness trends feature youthful images of sculpted success stories showing us their muscles and abilities. There are bodybuilding competitions (and yes, there are yoga competitions). There are muscle magazines and muscle cars. There are drugs and special diets designed to make them bigger, stronger, and "better." We are so enamored with muscle that we tend to perceive those without it as weak and insignificant, but this is what trends do. You're either in or out. We've created a muscle cult. Perhaps it's time to give some attention to the deeper parts. Relatively speaking, muscles are pretty superficial.

We cannot have healthy bones and joints if muscles steal the show. This is costly to overall health and vitality, and it's time for a more holistic approach. Everything changes when we repurpose the muscles and use them to condition the joints and bones. What about all the other tissues and systems that make up a body? What about the lymphatic system, the nervous system, and the vascular system? Instead of *only* exercising to make the muscles more prominent, what if we started using our muscles to make other tissues and systems healthier and more efficient?

Shape by shape and class by class, Avita consistently gives the muscles a higher purpose. It's a defining characteristic of the practice and a radical paradigm shift. If more people could make that shift and give their muscles the greater purpose of generating healthy joints and stronger bones, there would be fewer injuries, fewer surgeries, and fewer replacements. Many could exercise less and significantly improve their health, while those who dislike exercise might be inspired to do something so simple to care for their overall well-being. And they might all find a more peaceful presence, which is reason to smile more often.

WE BLAME THEM

There's a love/hate relationship to every dramatic story. We love muscles when we see them, but we blame them for just about everything. We stretch them, we poke them, we prod them, we stimulate them, we heat them, and we ice them. But it's not the muscles' fault. They are not the cause of their condition. Muscles can be chronically tight because of unresolved physical, mental, or emotional trauma, which means the therapy you seek for your muscles is best when it also includes a way to relax the nervous system and unwind the mind.

Take one specific body part, for example. Almost everyone thinks they have tight hamstrings. From low-back problems to hip pain, tight hammies are blamed for all kinds of issues. The most common phrase I hear regarding muscle pain is, "I have tight hamstrings." You don't, but your hip or lower back issue may make your hamstrings *feel* tight. You may have ankle or knee rigidity, signaling the hamstrings to contract and shorten as a protective mechanism. Your hamstrings could be "tight" because they are organized according to how you carry yourself and walk through life. They can often feel tight because they have been overstretched and are trying to recover. In short, they are "tight" not of their own accord but because your supercomputer brain has instructed them to be this way.

Rarely, if ever, are muscles tight or problematic alone. The restriction or problem is almost always elsewhere, and you can do harm by repeatedly trying to stretch muscles and targeting the wrong problem. Just because you can't touch your toes doesn't mean your hamstrings are tight! Give them some love. Just because you feel them approaching natural extension does not mean they are tight. The hamstrings are one of a few muscle groups in the body without a hard stop. Most other muscle groups have a physical limit where one body part bumps into another, which automatically limits extension.

There are a couple of others, but we don't think about testing them and pushing on them the way we do the hamstrings. How determined are you, for example, to bend your fingers back toward the top of your forearm? We don't because it doesn't look good. But many are determined to touch their toes or bring the forehead to the knees because it's elegant. It has oddly become a conventional measure of health.

Wouldn't fibers be susceptible to overextending or tearing if a muscle group evolved to have no natural limit? Without a firm limit, wouldn't the muscle be especially sensitive to excessive extension? Might it be programmed to err on a slight "tightness" for good reason? The hamstrings have to support the entire posterior side of the body from the knee to the pelvis and lower back. They have a job to do and don't benefit much from your meddling in it. Treat them kindly and focus on your ankles, knees, hips, and spine instead. Freeing these joints along with the tension in the nervous system will trickle up and down your body and bring lasting, youthful results. Your hamstrings will take care of themselves. Muscles adapt according to the health of the nervous system and the resiliency of the joints and tissues they move.

SIZE MATTERS NOT

Muscles appear more prominent only because of an increase in volume. Muscle fibers are specialized cells that cannot increase in number by dividing, as many other kinds of cells do. When you strength-train, the body's homeostatic mechanisms sense the increased workload and send the appropriate signals to the cells to handle the load, causing proteins to grow inside the cell. The result is a bigger muscle fiber.[40] But there is a cost to focusing attention on muscles alone. How does increased muscle mass affect the flow of blood? Does the heart have to work harder to get blood through dense tissues? What happens to the blood vessels and capillaries deep in the tissue? It may all adapt, but what happens over time if the bodybuilding stops? Do the blood vessels readjust as muscle mass decreases? What about the lymphatic vessels? What happens to oversized muscles with the inevitable atrophy that comes with age?

I don't know the answers to these questions, and I'm not raising them to induce controversy or fear. I think they are good questions inspired by a book called *Haywire Heart* by Lennard Zinn, Christopher J. Case, and Dr. John Mandrola. Their book explores the prevention and treatment of heart conditions in athletes like arrhythmia, atrial fibrillation and flutter, tachycardia, hypertrophy, and coronary artery disease. Many of these conditions are the result of over-exercising the heart, and the heart is a muscle.

How do we know our approach to fitness or health has our best long-term interest in mind? Look closely at the motivating factors. If you enjoy lifting weights or strength training, do it for the joy. Doing something you truly enjoy will often yield healthy results.

I've had bodybuilders in my classroom, and most of the older ones have degenerative problems. They have a different version of the same pain cycle that anyone can fall into. As joint movement becomes limited, problems like calcification, arthritis, and degeneration show up. They might go unnoticed because of the body's ability to bury problems, but hidden issues eventually catch up to us. As alternatives to medication and surgery, bodybuilders handle the pain like many others do by fortifying the joints with stronger muscles. Increasing muscle strength to "stabilize" joints is common but provides temporary relief at best. It misses the problem and "protects" it from true healing.

Although the "workout" is often enough to bolster the joints and ward off pain, its effects are fleeting. Many athletes take the same approach to pain management: If I strengthen my muscles, the pain will go away, and I can keep moving and playing my sport.

But pain, and injury, send a message. Maybe it's time to slow down and think about the ramifications of intensity. True humility is healing and powerful. It requires us to honestly examine the beliefs and values we assign to the body. Try as we might, the body cannot overcome thoughts of fear and lack. They remain in the mind, negatively impacting the body, until we identify and release them.

The muscles we are born with have a specific density, length, size, and mass that fit the body we came in with. We risk disorganizing the structure if we develop an agenda to grow, strengthen, or stretch them. Bones are not alluring or sexy, but they make up the important framework. And because we often believe that more is better, we tend to overdo, overuse, overbuild, and over-strengthen, unaware that we may begin to underuse the cartilage, bones, and joints. We erroneously think that if it looks good on the outside, it must be good on the inside. Don't be fooled: Large, powerful muscles can overshadow healthy joint function and potentially impede the intrinsic movement vital to joint health and longevity.

Which do you prefer, bigger muscles or healthy joints and bones? Which would best serve you for a lifetime? In Avita we don't do repetitions, nor do we use outer resistance—we have plenty built-in. The active shapes provide steady and complete muscle activation that utilizes and unwinds the *inner resistance* in the muscles, fascia, bones, and joints. It's lovely when it all works harmoniously together.

THE FOUR MUSCLE CHARACTERISTICS

Different tissues in the body have unique characteristics that enable specific functions. When these characteristics are violated, the tissues' ability to perform their given function breaks down or fails altogether.

Here are the four universally accepted characteristics of muscles:

- **Excitability:** Muscles are stimulated or "excited" by the nervous system.
- **Contractility:** Muscles contract or shorten to move body parts.
- **Extensibility:** Muscles release and lengthen.
- **Elasticity:** Muscles can return to their original, neutral state.[41]

Let's focus on the elastic characteristic of muscle. It is the one that is most often misunderstood. The encyclopedia Britannica defines elasticity as the "ability of a deformed material body to return to its original shape and size when the forces causing the deformation are removed. A body with this ability is said to behave (or respond) elastically." It goes on to say that there's a limit to how much stress a material can withstand before it undergoes permanent deformation (plastic deformation). This limit is called the elastic limit.[42] Rubber bands have elasticity, and so do tennis balls and even human skin.

Flexibility and elasticity are not the same. Elasticity is an adaptable quality where an object or material returns to its original shape after being altered. A rubber band is flexible *and* elastic by nature. As long as you stay within the confines of its characteristics—size, thickness, length—when you stretch a rubber band, it returns to its original length and shape. But if you pull it too far, too often, it will tear bit by bit and lose its elasticity. That's the stretch! When it happens, it loses the ability to return to its original shape and length.

Extensibility is also often misunderstood. It, too, is equated with "stretch," but it refers to the ability of a muscle to release. Make a fist and squeeze. The muscles on the palmar surface contract while the ones on the back of your hand and your fingers extend. Now, open your hand and expand your fingers. Can you see and feel the muscles change roles? Stretching can be a feeling, but it is not a characteristic of muscles.

To summarize the four characteristics, muscles are excited by an electrical stimulus from the nervous system, which causes them to either contract or extend. When the stimulus or action is over, the elastic characteristic of muscles allows them to return to their original length or state.

MUSCLES DON'T STRETCH

This point is important enough to add further emphasis. Muscles do what they are told to do. They don't release or extend unless the nervous system messages them to do so. It's not a matter of them being long or short, flexible or stiff. It's a matter of the neuro-stimulation being sent to your muscles. Each fiber within a muscle is either "on" or "off." There is never a partially contracted muscle fiber. When you move your hand toward your face to drink a glass of water, the biceps and the flexor muscles in the fingers and hand activate. But simultaneously, neurotransmission informs the opposing muscles to release and *extend*, allowing smooth movement to occur.[43] Nothing happens by accident. Every movement is managed, so when the subconscious messaging gets mixed up, as in disorders like MS and Parkinson's, the parts don't move the way we want them to.

Muscles don't stretch, they release.
Fascia is malleable and made to change.

Have you ever tried to stretch a piece of meat before cooking it? It's not stretchy. Even in a warm body, muscle tissue doesn't stretch. If it did, we would not be able to stabilize ourselves. We'd be "all over the place." The primary difference between a piece of meat and working muscle tissue is that muscles in a living body are innervated. Muscle is not stretchable tissue; it contracts and extends. When one muscle (the agonist) contracts, there's an automatic deactivating message sent to an antagonist to "let go" or "extend," which allows for coordinated movement. This is known as reciprocal inhibition, and Avita Yoga uses it to safely bring full movement to muscles and joints.[44] When a muscle is encouraged to extend beyond its relaxed limit, it is interpreted as a "stretch." Is it natural? Is it helpful? Is it necessary?

So, what causes muscle tightness? It's complex and could lead to questions about diet, hydration, stress, medications, and exercise habits, to name a few.[45] There are factors that include the nervous system and chemical contributors including hormones. We also know that muscle tissue and the fascia around it work hand in hand. Each adapts to support the other. With so many factors influencing muscle resiliency, are we creating a problem where it does not exist? The change we want in Avita Yoga targets the bones, joints, and fascia while asking for full contraction and extension of muscle groups. While you may feel stretchy sensation at times, we are not stretching. It's a safe and effective way to resolve restrictions and promote muscle tone.

RISKS OF TOO MUCH "STRETCH"

Fascia is malleable; muscles are not. What could happen if muscles are overextended or conditioned in a way that impedes their elastic ability to return to their original length of form? It's familiar but often overlooked knowledge that physically overextending muscle tissue results in small micro-tears. If repeated, the muscle may tear and repair again and again, resulting in a longer muscle with decreased elastic ability to return to its original form. Muscles must return to their original state to stabilize body parts and balance the body properly. Returning to our camping analogy, imagine a tent with a few slightly longer guylines. It will affect the integrity of the whole tent.

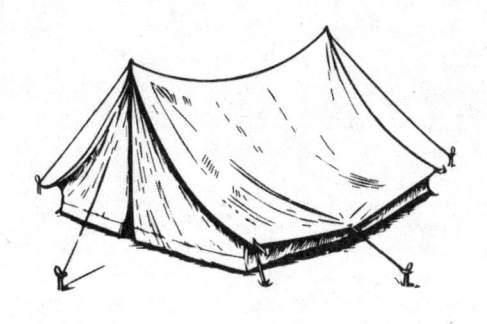

Here's an example I've seen in accomplished yoga teachers and students. If the hamstring muscles are overstretched, they lose their ability to stabilize the back of the pelvis. They attach to the sit bones, which are part of the pelvis. Overstretched hamstrings allow the pelvis to tip forward, inducing the lordotic arch in the lower back. The lower back arches, the sit bones rise, and the upper back flattens. Muscles between the shoulder blades compensate for "support" from above, creating fatigue. This compensation response leads to upper back and neck pain, while clearly, the cause is elsewhere. In constant lordosis, the lumbar spine loses its ability to flex over time because the hamstrings have lost their essential function.[46]

It's what we have come to recognize as "good posture."

Rather than building bulk or overstretching, we want the muscles to be healthy, functional, and supple. Targeting muscles for flexibility misses the problem, diminishes integrity, and often overrides stretch receptors that send feedback to the central nervous system. In Avita, we work from the bottom up and from the inside out. All the parts need to work together, so we use them *together* in our practice. As we experience the benefits of increased mobility and blood flow, the desire to stretch falls away. The more we target and resolve joint and fascial restrictions, the more supple and healthy the muscles become.

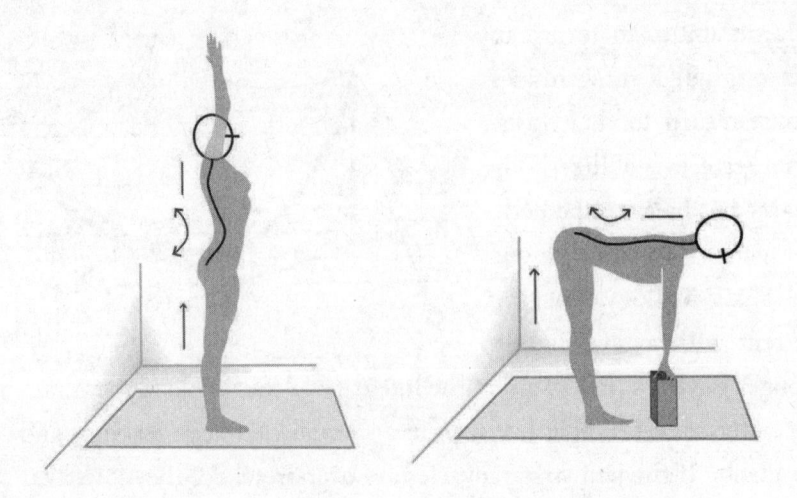

Left: Note the strong lordotic curve resulting from overstretched hamstrings. The pelvis spills forward and the upper back often flattens. The movement only becomes problematic when rules are applied to the body. Right: The pattern is compounded with repeated forward folding only from the hip while excluding lumbar flexion.

Finally, one of the observations I made in my youth that contributed significantly to the Avita approach to yoga is that I have never seen any animal stop and physically stretch their muscles before or after a run or high-speed chase. They pandiculate. Mammals share the same basic anatomical and physiological principles, and humans are the only mammals conditioned to stretch, which mostly came about in the 1970s.

There is much to say about pandiculation, and I recommend the article in the footnote from the Somatic Movement Center. Pandiculation is a full-body contraction of one group of muscles (agonists) that involves the simultaneous release or extension of a group of opposing muscles (antagonists). You'll see cats and dogs do it after a period of inactivity. Do you? It's a reset of the nervous system and happens for various reasons. But mostly, it feels good! It's what we are supposed to do when we wake up from sleep or a nap, and it's what we do in Avita at the end of most classes. Throughout the class, we respect the principles of natural pandiculation through reciprocal enervation discussed above. Pandiculation is very different than physically trying to stretch muscle tissue.[47]

WEAR, TEAR, AND TIME

There are consequences to overriding muscle characteristics and not listening to the body's feedback. It gets complicated. When muscles are extended beyond their limit, a feeling of soreness or tightness may follow. Watch for delayed onset of pain when the micro-torn muscle feels sore and stiff. This may not be the feedback you want, but if you get it, listen carefully. Overextending muscle tissue can result in a menacing issue that is slow to heal. We can get away with a lot in our youth, but patterns, habits, and self-imposed rules tend to catch up to us down the road.

Muscles produce the sensation of tightness as they recover from overextension and, because they feel tight, they are often targeted for *more* stretching. The feeling of stretching can become a drug that brings moments of relief along with a temporary high. Stretching movements and postures repeated in the same compensatory patterns hide the deeper issues while making the loose places looser. It's a massive paradigm in the yoga and fitness world where we impose outer mechanical characteristics and beliefs onto the body's inner workings. There is little in the outside world that mimics the body's inner workings. It is better to slow down, get clear on your motivation, and make sure you are targeting the parts that need it most.

Age is also a factor in muscle health since time has its way with *everything* in form. Have you tried to use a rubber band that's been in the junk drawer for a few years? Its characteristics have changed, and it won't perform as it once did. Similarly, muscles can tear and rupture if put to the test. Like any material, if you stretch a muscle too much, too often, it will have trouble returning to its original shape and condition.

The nervous system naturally restricts muscles around an injured area to minimize further damage and promote healing. This is the body's immediate response to trauma for damage control. It is a stabilizing phenomenon that is beneficial in the short term. However, unless the trauma is resolved, this "splinting" response goes from being an asset to a liability and can become chronic. In a sense, Avita takes us back in time to undo the harmful effects of trauma. We all have it; good things happen when we face it and unwind the past.

FLEXIBILITY VS. MOBILITY

There is a belief that mobility equals flexibility—and that flexibility equals comfort. I've fallen into this trap. Before Rolfing school, I believed a flexible body was better than a rigid one. I thought I could stretch and strengthen my way to better health. But beliefs obscure reality, and after many years of working with bodies and minds, I discovered that flexible people can experience pain and problems too.

Conversely, many who regard themselves as "stiff" are comfortable in their bodies. It's risky to jump to any conclusions. Let's discuss flexibility first.

As we have established, muscles get blamed for tightness but always behave according to the stimulus they receive. Where does it come from? In broad terms, we are each preprogrammed or "wired" with a particular constitution toward loose or tight. Some are born more flexible or rigid than others, but all are naturally drawn to activities in which they are competent. Of course, one's constitution alone does not govern one's interests, but it plays a significant role in one's probability of excellence and potential for injury in a chosen sport or activity. Contrary to popular belief, a certain degree of natural stiffness is needed for muscles to have a robust, springy quality.[48]

Hormones play a factor as well. They interact with the nervous system and influence where we land on the continuum between loose and tight. Boys often lose their inherent flexibility as they go through puberty. Women will sometimes lose flexibility when they go through menopause. Our "chemical soup" is affected by many things, including hormones, medications, foods, beverages, and our thoughts and feelings. It's easy to overlook these variables, compare ourselves to others, and jump to conclusions about our bodies and their capabilities.

We all come into the world with a certain degree of flexibility, which will vary over a lifetime according to the above-mentioned factors. As such, *flexibility* has to do with our hormonal and neurological programming and their effects on the muscles and other soft tissues. How else could we explain the fact that women tend to be more flexible than men? *Mobility* has to do with articulating joints and their range of motion. It has little to do with the muscles and much more to do with the restrictions and limitations in and around the joints.

Your physical parts may feel stiff and inflexible, but this feeling is a poor indicator of your ability to generate joint mobility and health. On the other hand, people with exceptional flexibility often feel tight because their muscles must work harder to support the body in simple daily activities. Their muscles are doing the job that their bones and joints should be doing. Is the problem in the structural components or in the nervous system? Either way, the solution is the same in Avita, because we use the muscles to target the bones and joints, which automatically reorganizes the nervous system.

Even if the shape does not "improve," our neurochemistry rebalances along the way. We get to stop looking for outer variables (people, places, things, and consumables) to influence our inner well-being. Our yoga practice challenges the structural and neurological patterns to reorganize the systems, tissues, and cells. Which comes first—the change in the structure or the neurochemistry behind it? Which is most important? It doesn't matter, because we aim for practical overall results that we can feel.

The body organizes itself according to the brain's interpretation of the feedback it generates. Flexible individuals who overdo—whether it be yoga, gymnastics, or dance—often feel tightness in the areas they repeatedly overstretch. Why? Because as we have already noted, overextended muscle tissue is continually trying to recover and return to its original shape. People with tight constitutions, on the other hand, avoid the movements almost entirely.

The benefits of any physical practice depend on how we use the feedback the body generates. If the goal is a physical accomplishment, the inner feedback will be considered a hindrance and avoided. This is ubiquitous thinking in high-level athletics. Aware of it or not, we avoid the painful, tight, and achy areas, and movements that provoke unpleasant sensations are off-limits. In contrast, the parts of the body that are loose and mobile tend to get more attention and action because they lead to physical success and are celebrated and rewarded. In short, flexible areas become more flexible and overused; tight areas get tighter and underused.

Avita Yoga brings this bias front and center. We teach the shapes in a way that exposes the tight areas *and* the loose areas. We can practice in a way that stabilizes overly mobile parts while bringing movement to the places that need it most. Where there's movement, there's health. Where there's stagnation, there's calcification. When we practice according to Avita principles, the body gets reorganized from the inside out. Movement is more fluid, and there are fewer aches and pains. Balance and agility improve, making us less prone to falls and injury.

Best of all, we learn to get out of the way. There is no manipulation in Avita. We don't need electrical wires and lights to give us "biofeedback." The response mechanism is built-in. All we have to do is listen to it and stop trying to eliminate the sensations we don't like. As we learn to *listen* and let the shape do the work, the body reorganizes itself, sometimes quite quickly.

THE SCIENCE OF "THE STRETCH"

I'll briefly describe the science behind muscle contraction and extension to support the discussion above. This is for the scientist within, and there are other valid theories about muscle contraction, but this is the predominant one.[49]

The sarcomere is the basic unit of contraction in the muscle fiber. As the sarcomere contracts, the overlap between the thick and thin myofilaments increases. As it extends, this area of overlap decreases, allowing the muscle fiber to elongate. Additional stretching places force on the surrounding fascial sheaths once the muscle fiber reaches its maximum resting length. As tension increases, the collagen fibers in the connective tissue align along the same force line. Stretching, at its best, encourages muscle fibers to release and extend to their fullest potential, which exposes fascial adhesions so they can be reorganized and resolved.

When muscle extends, a tiny proprioceptor called the muscle spindle measures the change and speed of the lengthening and conveys this information to the spinal cord. This is known as the *stretch reflex*. The more sudden the change in muscle length, the stronger the stretch reflex. The stronger the reflex, the stronger the muscle contraction. This essential function of the muscle spindle helps to maintain integrity and balance and to protect the body from injury. It's an automated function that happens in milliseconds and that we do not consciously control.

It constantly operates to keep us upright, balanced, and safe without thinking about it. It's designed to occur so quickly that sending the message up the spinal cord to the brain would take too long.

Have you ever felt like you were losing your balance, and the perfect group of muscles kicked in to bring you back upright? That's the stretch reflex in action. Believe it or not, many stretching programs use techniques to override this mechanism.

One less beneficial reason people hold a stretch for a prolonged period is to keep the muscle in an extended position. This habituates the muscle spindle and makes it less sensitive. It becomes accustomed to the new length and reduces its signaling. You can train your stretch receptors to allow greater muscle extension. But why? With specific training, the stretch reflex can be controlled so that there is little or no reflex contraction in response to a sudden stretch. While this type of control provides the opportunity for the most significant extension of muscle tissue, it misses the joints and can enhance the risk of injury.

The stretch reflex has both a dynamic and a static component. The static component persists as long as the muscle is extended. The dynamic component, which can be very powerful, lasts for only a moment and responds to a sudden increase in muscle length. The stretch reflex is a helpful protective mechanism that should be respected and not manipulated.

In Avita we don't warm up to help us accomplish more challenging positions. Warming up hides the problem and interferes with the most poignant feedback. The only "warm-up" is for the mind to relax and find its peaceful center, from which we seek to observe the body as a wholly neutral entity. The primary skill we learn in Avita Yoga is the discernment between pain and healing sensation.

In Avita, we work with the raw and unembellished body. We may "warm up" the mind by calming it down, but we do not warm up the body. With a hot or "warmed up" body, it's harder to find restrictions and easier to miss the deep healing compression bones and joints love.

MUSCLE AND JOINT PERSONALITIES

Each muscle and each muscle group has its unique quality of feedback. Muscles have proprioceptors to optimize movement and safeguard themselves, giving them unique "personalities." Many variables affect them, including their degree of leverage, their load, how often they are used, and whether or not they have had an injury.[50]

Joints also have unique qualities and characteristics. For example, those in the toes and feet can tolerate much more pressure than the joints of the fingers and hands, and for good reason. We walk on our feet, not our hands. Some joints house greater emotional sensitivity. Knees are particularly vulnerable and can bring up strong, sometimes fearful emotions when they are not working properly or become painful.

Then there are functional characteristics to consider. We can get by much easier with a bum ankle than a bum knee, for example, and so we'll tend to protect knees over hips and ankles because of their importance in daily life. Hips are big, stable joints buried in soft tissue, making them less sensitive than knees. We may not like having back pain, but it is less likely to stop us from doing what we love than knee or ankle pain. The shoulders carry the world, and while we can get around okay with shoulder problems, the pain is "close" and annoying. Since the neck and shoulders share muscles and nerve bundles, they are intimately related. That "pain in the neck" could result from a shoulder issue, and vice versa.

Notice the quality and character of feedback in muscles and joints as you practice and respect them. Thoughts, emotions, and physical sensations that surface along the way are part of the practice. It's all welcome, because it all resolves together. Now let's dive a little more deeply into this and learn how it relates to the nervous system.

CHAPTER 9

Our Unawareness of the Nervous System

We can describe feelings and sensations, but it's difficult to be aware of the nervous system itself, because it works behind the scenes. And yet, we need inroads to it because we aim for a calm nervous system and relaxed mind. Ironically, trying to work directly on the nervous system to get it to calm down can be counterproductive. It's almost impossible to target the nervous system and *make* ourselves relax.

Avita Yoga calms the nervous system as a by-product of practice, not because we target it and try to change it. To get the best results for the overall health of the brain and nervous system, we need to access it through the "back door." It's best if it doesn't know we are working on it, so this section of the book aims to inform you about what is going on behind the scenes to help improve the health of your nervous system, brain, and mind.

Avita will help balance and support your body regardless of your lifestyle. Steady compression on the bones and joints is remarkably soothing to the mind. It stimulates the parasympathetic nervous system. and in the long run, reorganizes the structure for better function.

Structural stability and resilience bring physical and emotional well-being. The bones are the deepest physical layer of the body. Reaching the bones is "profound work," which is why we take a slow, deliberate approach. But there is a "layer" beyond the bones—the nervous system. And herein lies one of the most important and beautiful revelations of Avita Yoga. *The bones are a direct path to the nervous system and mind.* There are millions of proprioceptors in the fascia around the joints, and they have much to tell us. These proprioceptors lead us to the problem where we hang out, observe, and wait for restrictions to release and blockages to unravel. We get closer and closer to ever-present calm by consistently removing the obstacles to it. We are reprogramming for inner peace.

Have you ever considered the possibility of *reorganizing* and improving the overall health of your nervous system? How would you do it? The way most of us think about boosting the health of the nervous system, which includes the brain, is to learn a new skill—solving puzzles like Sodoku or learning a new language. Others take up activities like pickleball, cycling, or something else that requires new dexterity. Your ability to learn an exciting new skill will come with more joy and ease if you unwind the old patterns and blockages along the way. In an Avita class, we aim to access the parasympathetic nervous system even in our active and sometimes demanding shapes. This helps us carry the calming effects of practice into our lives. We are rewiring our innate intelligence to access a calm presence. You will often hear me say, "there is a meditation in every shape". We are meditating, healing our bodies, and unwinding our nervous system for long-term benefit.

Instead of putting a new skill on top of an old one, consider undoing old, unhelpful patterns. The result is more clarity, less clutter, and healthier neurological connections. Is this different from the goal of meditation? Aren't we trying to gain peace and clarity? If not, why meditate? Avita Yoga is the best of both worlds. It's a moving meditation that resolves inner conflict and brings clarity to the mind.

NEUROPLASTICITY

Perhaps you remember the movie *What the Bleep Do We Know?* It conveyed one key concept: The mind can fall into a groove where the nervous system is hardwired into recurring and often destructive patterns. Synaptic responses are habituated, the body's chemical composition alters, and it becomes increasingly difficult to get out of the unhelpful groove and into a healthier, happier way. But we can change it for the better, and neuroplasticity is the buzzword for this resilient way of being. Neural networks can reorganize and function with greater efficiency.

Dysfunctional synaptic responses can be reprogrammed to become healthier and happier pathways. In a sense, neuroplasticity is the idea of getting unstuck at a neurological level.[51] Some say we can rewire ourselves to manifest a particular outcome for the body or author the life we want. I don't speak to that much because in my experience when I tried to manifest the life that I *thought* I wanted, it didn't work. It did not bring happiness. In fact, it led to struggle and pain and became another turning point in my life that had to be forgiven and released.

But I *can* talk endlessly about the miraculous benefits of getting out of my way and removing the obstacles to joy and peace of mind. I can speak to the madness of trying to manifest a life "I" want because it comes from the separate sense of self known as the ego. It is deluded into thinking it actually knows what it wants and can control its way to happiness by getting what it wants in form. I can talk at length about the miracles of changing my mind from the beliefs that uphold the separate self to a unified awareness of the one love we share. This book and the joy of sharing it would not be possible without the Guidance of Higher Love.

There's risk in trying to make the body flexible, but with a flexible mind, *wow!* Anything is possible. Our yoga should *improve* neurological flexibility. But too often, an agenda for a flexible, high-performance body can be a substitute for the mental and neurological flexibility required for true freedom. Are you a high performing athlete who dislikes the sport? Are you pushing for short term gains that come with long term costs? In his book, *Open*, Andre Agassi shares his disdain with the sport that made him wealthy and well known. Your performance may be high, but what about lasting inner fulfillment and joy? In constant pain, Andre ignored the feedback and paid the price to excel by listening to the inner voice of guilt spurred by familial pressure. Of course it was an essential part of his healing journey. Is pushing through pain a part of yours?

Slowing down and using Avita shapes to generate new neural pathways has a youthful effect on the body and mind. I've had this experience and heard it from students who say they feel sharper, happier, and more open-minded. It's what we expect from practice. We celebrate all the results.

I appreciate the idea of neuroplasticity because it suggests we are not seeking bodily flexibility and performance as much as mental resiliency. Avita requires you and your brain to rethink your approach to movement, and the results play out in typical everyday actions like putting on a T-shirt or walking up a flight of stairs. It all gets easier. In this way, Avita is an *undoing* that anyone can do. Putting a new skill on top of old patterning does little good. Would you buy a new computer and load the operating system and software from the old computer? Of course not. You want the complete upgrade.

Systemwide improvements to the body can also be made through cortical remapping, where parts of the brain that govern specific movements and actions are enhanced or rehabilited after injury or disease.[52] And it happens best when we stop trying to make it happen. The brain can relax during class because you don't know what shape or movement is coming next. We stop anticipating and drop into the sensation that points us inward to the present moment. The whole practice is designed to remove the "I know" mind from the equation so we can get out of our own way and let a better way come through.

My expertise in the nervous system ends here. The idea of neuroplasticity and the ability to rewire ourselves is helpful and will occur with time and practice. But I find it most beneficial to go beyond my brain and body for the healing power. Is this not what a *spiritual* practice is for? Awakening to the unified mind goes beyond neurology. You can measure brain waves, and scientists can measure synaptic responses. But our inner "movement" toward peace and happiness is immeasurable because it is an *experience* we're after, not a scientific calculation. What evidence do we need beyond an experience?

A MOBILE FOUNDATION

We don't usually think of foundations requiring mobility. Buildings would not last if the foundation kept shifting. Our bodies are different. Our balance is impaired if our joints lack the mobility to adjust. The vestibular system coordinates with millions of proprioceptors concentrated in the connective tissues around the joints, which relay information about movement and position to the nervous system and brain. The data and appropriate response are processed in milliseconds, and billions of neurons fire off up to fifty action potential messages per second.[53] This allows you to process your surroundings and generate the best action to catch yourself before you fall or stay upright and balanced on two feet in all you do.

If you stub your toe and trip, the message from your misstep originates in your toes, feet, knees, and hips, then goes to the spinal cord for processing, and then back to the body parts that need to move to prevent the fall—all without thinking about it. What movement feature is going to help you the most? Mobility. Anybody can attain this with practice.

CHAPTER 10

Our Ignorance with Connective Tissue

My training at the Dr. Ida Rolf Institute was the best yoga education I've ever had because it taught me about patterns and fascial restrictions. I remember thinking it should be a requirement for humans to learn these things about their bodies. It took a knee injury to get me into the Dr. Ida Rolf Institute. It took a hip injury to blend and apply the principles of Rolfing to yoga more deeply. I experimented with my body to see what worked. With students it was similar. I would put them in a shape, use my hands at times to help release fascial restrictions, and then ask them to stand up and walk. Did we get the results we wanted? No, let's try something else. It's feedback-driven and it's how Rolfers learn to unwind fascial restrictions and patterns. Fascia holds the issues and it's there we begin to look for lasting change.

Avita has evolved by applying well-known anatomical and physiological principles to yoga. Who doesn't want the most direct path to restore youthful mobility and movement? Who has time to waste? We know that much of the change comes from the connective tissue, so where do we find it? Conveniently, it's everywhere and concentrated around the joints, where the muscle attaches to the bone. Restrictions are made in these areas, meaning we get the most mileage by targeting them, and every Rolfer and myofascial therapist is aware of it.

The terms *connective tissue* and *fascia* are often used synonymously, and while I use them both, most anatomists would agree fascia is a subset of connective tissue. Facia is an immense, interconnected network of supportive material throughout the body. It's the shiny white stuff on an anatomical chart that tends to get cut away to reveal the "important parts," but fascia is essential. It holds things together and creates a vast matrix that shapes and supports the body.[54]

Fascia gets thicker and denser near the joints where tendons attach to bones. It is so seamlessly enmeshed that it's challenging to determine where muscle starts and bone begins. Fascia surrounds organs and offers both support and glide. It provides structure to the blood vessels and the lymphatic system. It supports nerves. It gives everything its shape, which is partly why our shape changes as we age. Collagen production, which slows as we age, is vital in fabricating fascia.

How is fascia produced? A multifunctional fibroblast cell synthesizes the extracellular matrix and collagen, creating the structural framework for other tissues, and plays a critical role in wound healing. Fibroblasts are the most common cells of fascia. Fibroblasts and fibrocytes are two states of the same cells, the former being the activated state; the latter the less active state, concerned with maintenance and tissue metabolism. Fibroblasts are the soft-tissue version of the cells that remodel bone and cartilage, which we discussed in chapter 4. Whether bone, cartilage, tendon, or ligament, we have a built-in capability to repair and reorganize. And it's all stimulated by compressive forces and how we align and use our bodies.

OUR IGNORANCE WITH CONNECTIVE TISSUE

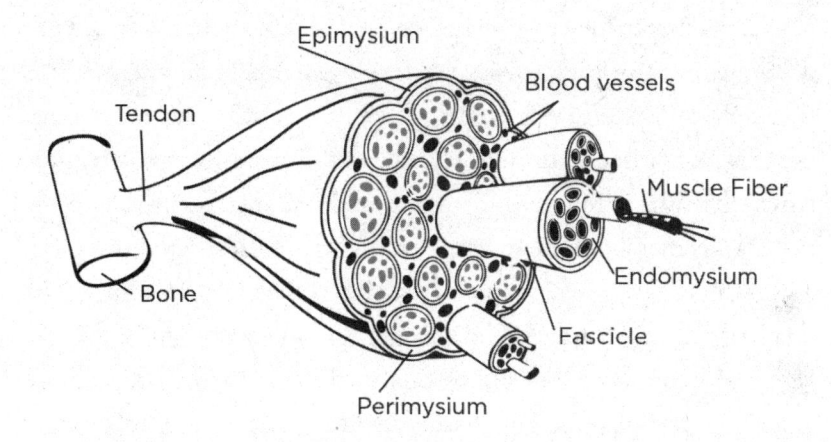

Notice the fascial covering on the three groupings of muscle tissue. From superficial to deep, we have epimysium, perimysium, and endomysium, all of which have changeable, adaptable properties that encase non-stretchable muscle tissue. The facial layers form a multidimensional matrix, seamlessly supporting and joining muscles with tendons, ligaments, and bones. Can you see the interconnectivity of it all?

FIBROBLAST

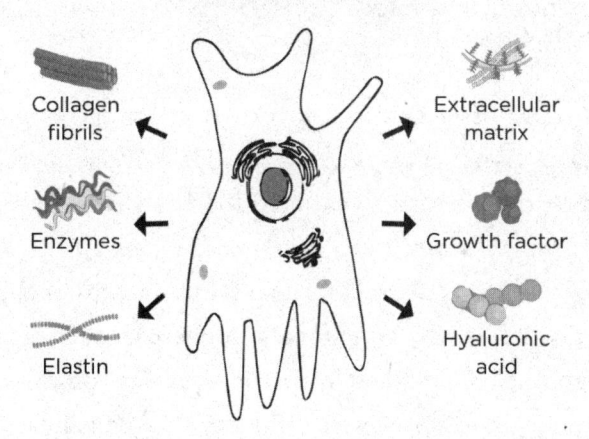

Check out this multitasker.

Let's jump up one categorical notch and talk about the two types of connective tissue: *collagenous or dense connective tissue* and *elastic or loose connective tissue*. As its name implies, collagenous connective tissue is comprised mainly of collagen. It provides tensile strength, which is why it is found in ligaments and tendons, but it also forms the fibrous membrane that wraps around the muscles, blood vessels, and nerves. It's strong, supportive, and has little need for an elastic quality.[55] Elastic connective tissue, on the other hand, has less collagen and consists primarily of elastin. Imagine that. Much more adaptive, elastic connective tissue creates a vast matrix to support cells that form tissues, store fat, and support the body's organs.[56]

What is fascia, and what does it do?
Fascia makes up our cellular matrix, our architecture. It binds and supports. It slides, glides, and reduces friction. It's rigid, formable, and adaptable. It contains nerve endings that communicate with the brain. It's the largest sensory system in the body. It's the most ubiquitous tissue in the body. It transmits force. It aids with wound healing.

Connective tissue contains a base substance called *mucopolysaccharide*, a lubricant that helps the fibers slide over one another. It also has bonding characteristics that hold the fibers together in bundles or strands, which is why it can develop adhesions.

Being everywhere, fascia forms a three-dimensional matrix of the body, which is why an anomaly in one part can lead to problems in another. Combined with the countless proprioceptors it houses, we begin to see why the problem and the pain are rarely in the same place.

CARTILAGE—PREFERABLE, BUT OVERRATED

Nature uses specialized cells to form tissues with specific functions in the body. Cartilage is one such fantastic tissue. It's denser than bone but softer and more resilient. It is found in various degrees of pliability and density in joints between bones, in the rib cage, the ear, the nose, the elbow, the knee, the ankle, the bronchial tubes, and the intervertebral discs.[57] In Avita Yoga, we are primarily concerned with the articular cartilage found on the ends of bones in joints like the fingers, knees, and hips, as well as the fibrocartilage that makes up the meniscus of the knee and the intervertebral discs of the spine.

Articular cartilage has a remarkably smooth, dense, and resilient glass-like quality, and we would all love to have a lifetime supply of it. Unfortunately, it usually doesn't last long if there is imbalance or toxicity within the joint space. Many have lost cartilage through degeneration and resorption to the point that some joints are "bone on bone." Cartilage is lovely, but if it resorbs, I believe that along with a clean diet, kind, consistent pressure can smooth and densify the bone where there was once cartilage. Lifestyle may change slightly, but you get to keep your original parts if you are willing to maintain them. While there are no studies to support this, I'm relying on the science mentioned earlier, my own experience of bone on bone in my neck, and the testimony from students who have improved mobility and reduced pain knowing they had bone on bone situations.

Fibrocartilage is found in the intervertebral discs of the spine and the meniscus in the knee, and functions like an adaptive cushion. Its spongelike nature allows it to absorb fluid, providing fibrocartilage with shock-absorbing properties. Fibrocartilage relies on consistent compression and decompression to cleanse itself and maintain resiliency. However, if the cartilage is resorbed and no longer exists in the knee, the same compressive forces will aid in remodeling and sustaining bone health while cleansing the fluid within the joint space.

Cartilage resorption can occur in any particular joint and may be painful in certain positions. But what is the cause of resorption? Is it an imbalance in the joint? Arthritis? Overuse? Aside from systemic factors like diet, smoking, and autoimmune issues, all of these ailments could stem from not giving the bones and joints the pressure they need to thrive. And the lack of cartilage does not make pain a certainty. Bone-on-bone refers to a condition where cartilage is absent in a joint and may or may not be accompanied by pain.

Research indicates that up to 31 percent of individuals over fifty may have radiographic evidence of knee osteoarthritis but not report any pain.[58] Similar trends have been observed in other joints such as the hips and hands.

Avita shapes do not assume that there is always an ample supply of cartilage in every joint. We work with what we have. We listen to the feedback, adjust the pressure accordingly, and practice consistently. Whether it's cartilage or bone, as long as it's not profoundly deformed and degenerated, practice can restore health and function to the joint. If the joint is in intermediate to advanced stages of degeneration, then it will take more practice in specific shapes, but don't fight it. There is a place and time for surgical replacement. Diet and lifestyle changes play a big part in the recovery of a joint at this stage. I often prescribe three to four additional shapes to practice daily for students that fit this profile. Despite periodic pain and decreased range of motion, many live a happy life and choose against a surgical repair. Naturally, all of these factors influence the exercise we engage in as part of our overall health journey—the topic of our next chapter.

CHAPTER 11
Exercise Redefined

Exactly what falls under the umbrella of *exercise*? My definition is simple: That which is challenged improves. Is that not the premise of exercising? I know there are many reasons to exercise. But fundamentally, most exercise so that something, usually muscle, gets more robust and more efficient. And because our time and energy are important, let's be very clear on *what* we exercise and *why*.

In Avita, we challenge the bones and joints to stimulate physiology that cleanses and remodels joints while making our bones stronger and denser. And because we use the muscles to do this, they are toned and released along the way. But we also exercise the heart and vascular system by *kindly* challenging them without requiring the heart to work faster. We do many shapes with legs up the wall and elevated arms to fortify the lymphatic system. We activate muscles by using them to release binding restrictions—all this and more while reorganizing the nervous system to operate more efficiently.

As your ability to target bone and joint health grows, you can relinquish the more superficial goals of losing weight, looking better, and getting fit. Set the goal for peace and use Avita for healthy bones and joints, and the secondary goals will fall into place with less effort.

Most people don't like to exercise, and I'm happy to say Avita is *not* a traditional form of exercise. Slow down, go deeper, and heal. Give all your activities a healing purpose, and all becomes "yoga."

THE NEED TO MAINTAIN WHAT YOU GAIN

Here's more reason to be careful about what, how, and why we exercise. As discussed earlier, we are enamored with "muscle beauty" and what we can achieve with them. But in a world of extremes, we can easily trade health for fitness and guilt ourselves into becoming something we are not. As bodies in form, we may desire a particular look that implies health, yet fitness and health are *not* the same. We assume that if exercise is good, more is better.

Your gains should be easy to maintain—for life. If not, you may be overexercising. It also helps to minimize outer feedback and go by how we feel. We get obsessed with a physical goal and then give up because what we see in the mirror doesn't match the (unrealistic) image we hold. Some appear visually fit yet are unhealthy on the inside. Others are healthy but don't portray the "fit look." Again, how do you feel? What can you gain and sustain with ease?

Sometimes, the questions we ask are more important than the answers we think we already have. We've discussed the risks of manipulating the body into something we believe is valuable. Going deeper, I might ask, "What motivates me to manipulate myself?" It's almost always a form of guilt and fear that hides the true Self, innocent and whole. Is your need for bigger, stronger, skinnier, faster a substitute for unwavering self-acceptance? If personal goals and dictates work against us, wouldn't it be wise to give up these limiting thoughts to access the true Self, the part of the mind that *always* has our best interest at heart?

Can we improve anything in form without the need to maintain it? Whatever we don't maintain degrades and falls apart. Incidentally, this test tells us what's real or not. Only the changeless is eternal and real. We won't find the changeless in an ever-changing world, which is why our yoga must include our thoughts and always point us inward to our timeless reality.

Whether a bridge or a bicep, anything we build in the world of form must be maintained; if not, time and gravity get the best of it. If we want something to last and be easy to maintain, let us be thoughtful about what we build. While nothing lasts in time and space, operating sustainably and simply can reflect our timeless truth.

The means and the goal are conjoined. We cannot know peace by fighting for it. We must *practice* peace to learn it. Similarly, we cannot lead wasteful lives and expect the fruits to last. The yoga we do must work for a lifetime to have sustainable results. Going for the bones, the joints that join them, and a peaceful mind feels sustainable. Using the muscles to make stronger bones and joints may not increase muscle size, but it *will* create tone and improve circulation. It may not make you "stronger," but it will remove the barriers to strength like arthritis, degeneration, and other aches and pains. You'll *feel* stronger. Avita will help you maintain mobility and balance, which become our greatest physical assets as we age. Avita Yoga can be practiced anytime, almost anywhere, and at any stage of life. Yes, I've had students in their nineties in the classroom. If there is body weight lost through Avita Yoga, it is not because we try to burn calories; it's because we release the thoughts and habits that hold the weight. It opens the heart and mind to new and better choices.

HEALTH OR FITNESS—WHICH DO YOU WANT?

We now know that health and fitness have become synonymous with youth and beauty, but health has nothing to do with those attributes. It's become so divided that the "fit minority" does most of the exercise. Meanwhile, the rest believe they have already failed because they can't do what it takes to be "fit and healthy." Can you see the dilemma?

We believe we can only benefit by "exercising" intensely. Consequently, many burn out or decide they won't succeed. Some stop before they start. Avita sets a much different tone. It is for all: for the inflexible and the flexible, for those weary of the need to force or who dislike exercising, for any who have pushed their bodies hard in their early, "indestructible" years and wish to reclaim a sense of youth in their later years. Avita is for those who want a better way regardless of their years.

Avita Yoga is not a sport. It's not something to get better at. It's not something used to impress yourself or anyone else. Do you consider it an accomplishment to brush your teeth or take a shower? Yoga is hygiene for the body and mind. Are you tired after a day of work? Instead of grabbing a drink, put your legs up the wall. Were you feeling sore and tight after that hike? Restore your hips with *sukhasana*. You'll soon learn more about that beneficial shape. But how about trying a simple variation on it now?

— LET'S PRACTICE —

Half Sukhasana:
Seated in a chair with both knees bent and your feet flat on the floor, place your right ankle on the left knee. Relax your lower back, slump into your chair, and maintain for about thirty seconds. You may feel rigidity in and around the right hip. If the sensation is strong, maintain the shape sustainably for ninety seconds to two minutes, and repeat on the other side. If the sensation allows, relax your head and slowly curve forward. Welcome any stiffness in your lower back and adjust according to the sensation in your right hip. Don't make it too stretchy in the outer part of the hip and upper

thigh. We respect the muscular limit and let the yoga occur in and around the hip joint. Maintain for ninety seconds to two minutes, slowly raise back up, and repeat on the other side.

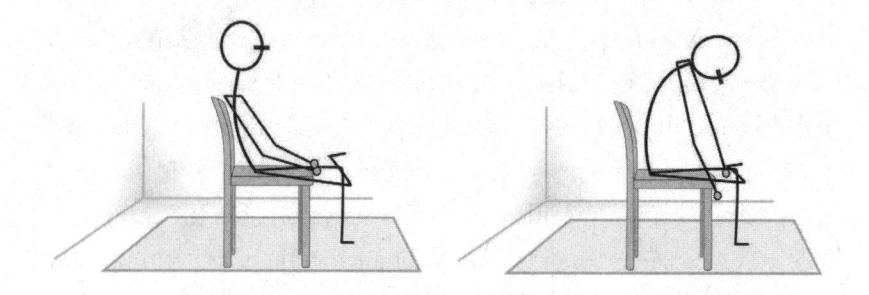

Scan the QR code to access Let's Practice video:

Are you getting the idea that the pursuit of fitness is dramatically different than the pursuit of health? Deciding on the proper health or fitness path can be confusing and intimidating. So, see if there are fitness demands you could do without. Instead of adding, what could you remove from your weekly schedule to feel better? The first two or three things that come to mind are worth considering. Should I add more responsibility or remove a stressor? More of anything is rarely, if ever, better in the long run. And we're in it for the long run. Perhaps it's time to reevaluate our cultural fitness goals.

Next, decide if you want to be healthy or fit. A gentle decision for health removes a lot of fear and guilt. The moment the "more is better" voice rears its ugly head, we push back. We can compete for an image we deem fit, but we cannot force health. Let peace be part of your goal for lasting health—it will begin when you decide to prioritize it.

Lastly, see if your short-term goals support your long-term goals. We plan for health by practicing for it here and *now*. Relinquish activities you are "supposed" to do or don't like. Why? Because if you don't like it, it won't work. You're out of yogic alignment when there is a discord between your thoughts and actions. Have you ever seen someone running or exercising who looks miserable? Think back to high school PE class and the students who did not want to be there. Maybe it was you? At times, it was me. Guilt and fear may push you in the short term, but they are unhealthy, deceitful motivators. Do the things you love and let Avita support them. Guidance will come naturally, and decisions about what is helpful or not will be made clear.

THE PROBLEM WITH DOING TO GET

We like to get better at what we're good at. It's logical, and it builds self-esteem. Getting better at something makes us feel good about ourselves. But let us go deeper: What could you get better at that would serve you forever? See—I told you we're in it for the long term.

Some of the most "accomplished" among us are often the most adamant about excelling. It's ironic, and while we hold this kind of performance in high esteem, it flirts with dangerous territory. It's a trap and can become downright cultish when we self-identify with anything of the body or outer world around us—whether it's a career, an athletic skill, a perfect set of abs, and so on. And when the day comes when the defining thing or activity is taken away, we're faced with the question we're most afraid to ask: *Who am I? Who am I without _____?*

Fill in the blank, let it go in your mind, wait for intuitive guidance, and keep doing the things you love, but don't let them define you. The sooner we release these binding chains, the sooner we can get to the Source of fulfillment and let it guide us in all we do. This is the yoga of a lifetime.

The attraction to specialized activities is often a delay tactic for peace and the source of many joint problems. Repetitious movement is not necessarily the issue. Specialized activity omits other vital movements that test the full range of motion necessary for joint health. No matter how accomplished we are at our job or activity, if we don't expose the joints to the more significant movement they crave, problems occur. Imagine the pattern in the hips for a professional cyclist, the knees for runners, the shoulders for swimmers, the lower back for truck drivers, and the neck and upper back for computer programmers and dentists. Where is the neuroplasticity if we repeat the same movements and thought patterns day in and day out?

In the conventional world of yoga and fitness, the push for bodily improvement can override the healing power of now by projecting a desired outcome into the future. There are often long-term ramifications for those who persist as they make demands on their bodies to perfect poses and movements under the guise that "once I get it right, all will be well and good." With Avita, we need *not* advance the shape to get results and feel better. We cannot push our way to health and mobility any more than we can demand our way into peace. *I can do it* becomes: I already have it, now let me realize it.

It's like making money without following your heart. You may advance the shape or pose, but at what cost? You may make money in a job you don't like, but is it worth sacrificing happiness? Pushing the pose is like serving wine before its time. The shape will evolve as it is supposed to—when it's ready, as the barriers dissolve. Ego demands, "Do something!" The healed mind says, "Relax, follow your heart, and the means will be provided." Urgency interferes with loosening and releasing our thoughts of doubt and fear. Wait, watch, and observe. The solution is at hand.

Specialization is not limited to sports. Our lives have become compartmentalized partly due to society's desire for efficiency. The more we adjust our surroundings to make life easier, the more we limit and specialize our movements. Perhaps the least specialized way of living is closer to nature, where we use the body in various ways to thrive, not just survive. For these reasons, I like practical, everyday movements like gardening, cleaning, fixing things around the house, landscaping, and the occasional bike ride, hike, or long walk. The body does well with variety, but if you're not accustomed to these things, pace yourself. Slowly take on natural, demanding movement, and have fun doing it.

Aging would be utterly hopeless if it didn't include the means and possibility of becoming something beyond the body. Wisdom is timeless because it is laced with acceptance, forgiveness, kindness, all-inclusiveness, and love. Wisdom is what we want because it transcends time, and it would be foolish to wait on time for it. Purpose is everything.

CHAPTER 12

The Cycle of Pain

CYCLE OF PAIN

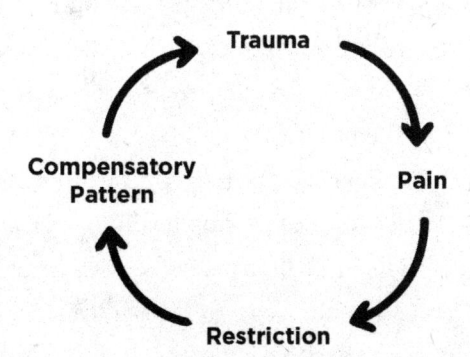

Trauma → Pain → Restriction → Compensatory Pattern → (Trauma)

The cycle of pain is put in motion by some form of trauma, whether physical (limiting movement), mental (limiting thoughts and beliefs), or emotional (limiting feelings). Each impacts the others and obscures the source of the problem. It's what the ego does best. Regardless of the source, pain produces a restriction, and we adjust our movement to compensate for it. These compensation patterns, are usually subconscious and lead the mind to believe that it is experiencing additional trauma, which is reinterpreted as pain.

The cycle continues, and the ruts get deeper. For example, a fall that traumatizes a hip brings pain. The pain produces a compensatory pattern, such as a limp, which exacerbates the problem and leads to lower back issues. Now, another part hurts and complicates the pattern. The cycle is thus kept in motion, and we keep chasing the pain and blame genetics or time for the symptoms we try to eradicate.

Regardless of the source, trauma sends percussive forces through the body, to which it continually reacts in a constant effort to heal amid an ongoing crisis. When we carry on as usual, it's chaotic on the inside, even if only at a subconscious level. We get good at pushing the problem down to keep moving on. Unless we get to the cause and unwind it, the body will never stop trying to heal as a response to the memory of the trauma. You bounced up after that fall on your bicycle when you were eight, but did the hip ever stop trying to mend? Where else did the percussive forces go? You may not remember it, but the body does.

An emotional incident long ago could be limiting movement and clarity today. When does a tree stop healing the scar of someone who carved their initials in it? Don't we all have a little PTSD from something traumatic? It's our yoga to find and unwind so we can row, row, row our boat merrily down the stream. In yogic terms, we're all healing from the frightening belief we separated from our Source. As a thankful nod to Dr. Freud, you could say we *all* have a little separation anxiety. Fortunately, yoga joins.

Instead of listening to the inner voice and getting the memory up and out, we tend to avoid the pain and push it down. We do what feels "good and right" according to our past conditioning. But to heal, we must interrupt the pain cycle; otherwise, we keep putting Band-Aids on problems made manifest by recurring dysfunctional patterns. But first, let's look deeper into the cycle of pain so we know what *not* to do, because the unhealed mind is impatient and always wants a quick fix.

FIX-IT MODE

When we want something fixed, we tend to rely on outer resources. Isn't that what you do when you discover a leak in your roof? "Outer" people and resources can be helpful—even necessary—and there have been many in my journey. But I'm keen to the temptation to over-rely on them. Injuries and issues have led me to all kinds of helpful people and insights. Still, the key has been to use the problem to look deeper within myself *as* I look to others for help. The answer is never "out there," but there are people *out there* who are predestined to help you the same way you and I are predestined to help others. I think of it as Divine Providence, and your/my/their current position in life is absolutely perfect to accept a healing function. It's how Avita evolved into my life, and it's how it finds its way into the lives of those it's meant to help.

Sometimes Avita is part of the solution, and sometimes it seems to *be* the solution. Regardless, we get the best results when we let the unwanted symptoms guide us deeper into our hearts and minds. What does that mean? It means we don't let fear be the guide, we don't skip steps, and we don't give our healing power to an outer authority. We welcome everyone into our healing as we hold space for theirs. In spite of outer appearances, we are all here to heal and imagine the outcome when we begin to accept our divine function.

Accept your role as a healer, and people will appear to help you heal. We cannot heal alone. A better way is at hand if we can step back and let it be shown to us. It could include conventional medicine, PT, massage, or yoga. Anything can be a piece of the puzzle, which means it's not just what we do but *how* we get there.

Do you remember watching the movie, *Groundhog Day*, where Phil the weatherman (played by Bill Murray) was caught in a time loop? No matter how hard he tried to impress and fix the situation, he couldn't obtain the goal of attracting Rita. But what if one of his manipulations worked? The goal in form would be attained without slowing down and doing the inner work that led to miraculous results. He was healed as he changed his mind about the situation that was causing enormous pain. Never again would he drop into that fearful state of wanting an outer result that met his needs because it was too painful.

This is the path we want, where the inner journey of changing the mind, healing, and joining brings worldly effects that are brighter and better than we could ever accomplish alone. *Groundhog Day* is a beautiful portrayal of "no accidents." You can see how every moment is a moment to choose again and learn that love (and nothing else) heals. Whatever is destined to be truly helpful comes from love.

To "fix" implies that something is broken. It's human nature. When we experience pain or discomfort, we *feel* broken, and we want the problem fixed so we can get back on the wagon and do the things we enjoy. In truth, you cannot be broken, but you can *believe* you can be broken. And you'll keep telling the story to prove it until the end of time, which will come, but why wait? Don't be duped by the delay tactic. Defense is an attack against the truth, which keeps it hidden from you. Next time you're in a coffee shop, sit back, enjoy your drink, and listen to the defenses disguised as stories safeguarding the fragmented and broken self.

Fixing objectifies and separates; healing joins and unifies. The former puts me in charge, while the latter lets healing come to and through. This yoga is about getting out of the way and undoing our resistance to true healing.

An Avita teacher can guide you into the shapes and the timing that remove resistance and move *you* toward a healed state. They can hold the container so you can get closer to the problem where it can be resolved. Snap judgments and reactions may pop us to the quick-fix surface, but we smile and gently return, willing to go deeper, where our peaceful center is waiting to be known.

POSTURE

There is no bad posture, and going for "good posture" often leads to problems down the road. The only good posture is the one you already have. It's the one you walk through life with. Posture is like art. The only "bad" art is that which we determine to be bad. If we see art as the artist's expression, there is no bad art. Posture, too, is an expression. To understand the art, it helps to know the artist. To understand posture, it's helpful to know the story behind it, which can help release past conditioning that formulates our judgment about what's good or bad.

We have been taught to strive for "correct posture" and buy in to the rationale for why it's correct and proper. Like diets, there are countless opinions on posture and what it means to have a good one. If we get stuck in our beliefs and how we hold ourselves, we unwittingly build our lives around them and defend them as part of our identity. Postural attitudes often originate in childhood when an authority figure demands a particular way of being in the body. These seeds are planted early, but instead of bearing fruit, they become unwanted weeds in the garden. Why? Because the best postural intentions can become holding patterns that limit natural, healthy movement.

Suppose you have subscribed to one of the many beliefs about proper posture and have been holding yourself in this manner either consciously or unconsciously. If so, you have probably developed both structural and psychological patterns. It's okay to let them go. As a child, I was quiet and contemplative, and, like everyone else, my body reflected my thoughts. I had a forward-head posture and was probably not as attentive as my dad wanted me to be. He often told me to hold my shoulders back, which put one pattern on top of the other. At age twenty-nine, prompted by my severe knee injury, I became a model in the first advanced Rolfing training. In a session, after working on my neck and shoulders, the teacher said to me, "Drop your shoulders and let them hang like a coat on a hanger." *What? You must be kidding*, I thought. *My dad told me to hold them back*. I was stunned. I heard this teacher clearly, but I wanted to argue with him. Oh yeah, I realized, my defenses are an attack against the truth. My spiritual practice served me well, and this was a turning point in my life that initiated my decision to become a Rolfer. It marked the beginning of a lot of undoing. Thank you, Advanced Rolfer Jan Sultan.

My dad's intentions were good. But no matter how well intended the advice, once it becomes a rule, it's only a matter of time before what was once helpful becomes a deeper problem. We must watch our enthusiasm for rules because they lead to control of self or others, and control comes from fear, which leads to devastation and separation. Bodily rules and lasting freedom cannot coexist. Rules lead to rigidity. In Avita, our only rule is *no rules*. When we let peace be our inner guide, it's impossible to "go wrong." What good ever comes from letting fear be the guide? This commitment comes through in the teacher training, where we learn not to correct but only to support and provide guidance toward healing sensation. What a gift.

Any fool will make a rule, and any fool will mind it.
—Henry David Thoreau

Adjusting how you walk or sit can reduce pain. Still, if that adjustment is made permanently without getting to the underlying problem, it's only a matter of time before it becomes problematic. When we hold and protect, the movement and our lives get narrower. We can't *hold* ourselves into freedom any more than we can *protect* ourselves into health. We must undo the barriers to movement and health. This was another golden nugget in my Rolfing training. Instead of imposing a new pattern to "right" a perceived wrong, *undo them all*. The result comes from an unwinding process to gain the freedom and health you are meant to have.

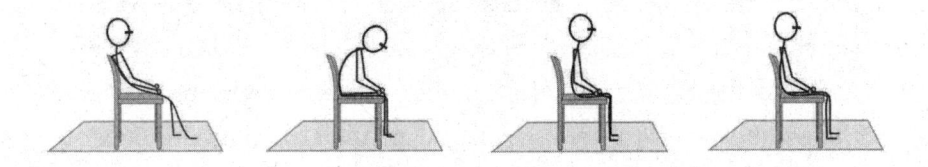

All of these ways of sitting are fine. Make any of them a rule, and it will become a problem. If adhered to, one "proper way to sit" will eventually limit healthy movement. Why not encourage children to sit in lots of different ways? And why not include ourselves in the freedom and fun too?

To delve a little more deeply into this important subject, the "proper posture" is a by-product of self-imposed beliefs that can become part of one's identity. To varying degrees, posture is "who we are" and, thus, the way we *hold* ourselves and present ourselves to the world. Any "improvement" to our presentation will eventually become a new problem. We cannot find freedom and joy by putting one pattern on top of another. We learn to hold ourselves in many ways: stiff, loose, uptight, upright, upstanding—oppressed, depressed, or debilitated. Do we not *hold* our bodies as a reflection of our deepest thoughts and beliefs? And while the body has no power over the mind, it feels like it does. Like any behavior change, changing the body or its posture is a substitute or quick fix for the deeper work. It's our yoga to *awaken*. Use your feelings to show you the thoughts and beliefs behind them, and let go of those that work against you. No one has to know you're doing it. Everyone will want to smile with you. As we change the mind, the body follows.

Naturally, the spine is the target of an unlimited variety of postural beliefs and demands. But at a fundamental level, there are only parts that move and parts that don't, and holding a special posture impedes the movement necessary to keep the spine healthy. When vertebrae stop articulating with one another, circulation is limited, and the calcification/degeneration process accelerates. Where there is movement, there is health. Avita Yoga facilitates movement throughout the spine by applying healing pressure to the parts that don't move while stimulating the body's natural physiology to restore health. The intellectual questions of "why" and "how" are far less important than the *experience* of freedom. We aim for enough mobility throughout the body to maintain joint movement. We want numerous ways to live, work, play, rest, and *be* in our bodies—for a lifetime.

In sum, the perfect posture is ever-changing and adaptable. Regardless of your chosen position, the ideal posture is the one that puts you in the most comfortable and efficient relationship to gravity with the least amount of effort.

COMPENSATION PATTERNS

My Rolf Movement® teacher, Vivian Jay, would often say, "The way you walk across a room is the way you walk through life."[59] What does our walk say about us? How does a person's lifestyle influence the way they walk? What parts move? Which parts are stuck? What's being carried forward from the past? It's helpful to bring the pattern to the light of our awareness and use it to unwind. We can each become self-healing detectives to find, identify, and gently resolve the patterns, our "ghosts" from the past.

In Avita, we use the shapes to work backward through time. The shape brings up a limitation that can bring up a memory. Both are welcomed, loosened, and released. Little by little, the past is undone. We want clarity on the patterns and how we walk through life. How do my thoughts limit me? What is favored? What parts are avoided? Is there a limp? What parts of the spine are stuck?

Because we *become* the pattern, we can't see it. The usual workout and fitness routines won't reveal it and, worse, can reinforce it. Even certain styles of yoga can reinforce the pattern when we omit the internal feedback and "go for" a particular pose. The loose parts get looser, and tight places remain hidden from awareness. It can be helpful to have an outside eye make an observation, but it's not necessary. Avita shapes and sequences address the patterns from the inside out.

Compensatory patterns manifest when physical blockages or mental constraints unconsciously push us toward a "path of least resistance." Hidden from awareness, it happens slowly over time. For example, a shoulder mishap brings pain, which limits range of motion, and after enough time, it becomes difficult to wash your hair with the affected arm. Instead of moving sustainably and consistently into the blockage, the path of least resistance—favoring the use of your other arm—increases the risk of a frozen shoulder. A hip problem turns into a benign limp, but the limp impacts the other hip and lower back. As time passes, everything organizes around a pattern, and scar tissue is laid down to support it. If enough time passes, the physical compensation gets wired into the nervous system, making it a hardware and software issue. No problem: We address them slowly and allow time in Avita shapes to unwind the nervous system and issue in the tissue. They are one and the same. When we address them simultaneously, we get the best results.

Sometimes problems originate in one body part and appear later in another. For example, a shoulder restriction can start in the hands or fingers. A wrist injury can unconsciously compromise routine activities like typing, holding a steering wheel, or cooking dinner, eventually impacting your shoulder. Years later, when the neck starts to complain, we assume that the pain and the problem are in the same place. The neck may need work, but it is not the source of the problem, so we must follow the pattern and go back through time to lift the original blockage (the wrist injury) to gain lasting results.

Finding the road less traveled takes gentle commitment and practice. If we think we know the answer, we're probably wrong, so we have to let it come to us by releasing our preconceived notions. It's poetic and abstract, but it works.

Be vigilant for harmful patterns. Loosening and releasing your thinking can become so fulfilling that at some point, we naturally devote our lives to the inner undoing. In this way, we are *all* saints and sages in training.

RESTRICTIONS, BLOCKAGES, AND ADHESIONS

There are differences, but I use these terms *restrictions*, *blockages*, and *adhesions* interchangeably when I teach. Why? Regardless of the limitations, we address them the same. We bump into them and spend time with them so they can release, remodel, and dissolve.

I cover the differences in more detail in our teacher training, but a basic understanding can benefit anyone who practices Avita. The terms have various definitions in the medical world. This is how I use them.

Restrictions form in the soft tissue around the joint. They are the earliest form of limitation resulting from unresolved trauma. Restrictions can result from compensation patterns and, in turn, reinforce them. They are an active part of the pain cycle mentioned earlier. Ultimately, we aim to catch and resolve restrictions before they become blockages.

While some **blockages** are congenital, they commonly form over time due to unresolved restrictions and movement patterns. Because restrictions and patterns reinforce blockages, the yoga that resolves them is the same. It may take a little longer, but bone can be remodeled along with fascial reorganization.

A blockage within the joint can present as tears and deformations, advanced arthritis, calcification, or stenosis. It can also result from adaptations in the cartilage and bone caused by repetitive movement patterns. For example, a cyclist's movement reshapes the hip joints, making a groove in the articular surfaces through repetitive motions. The result is limited internal and external rotation of the hips, which can lead to degenerative problems down the road. If caught soon enough, a blockage like this can be remodeled, and cycling can continue for life.

Restrictions are not limited to the articulation of bones and joints. They can also be found within the abdomen and thoracic cavity. When movement is limited, **adhesions** form between the internal organs, more commonly known as viscera. Joints have mobility. Visceral organs have motility. Again, where there is movement, there is health.

What could cause adhesions around the internal organs? Lack of movement of the spine. If the lumbar spine is stuck, the abdominal organs won't get the compression, push, and pull that "massage" them into a slippery, gliding movement against themselves. Rock-hard abs, as well as excessive abdominal fat, can limit and insulate the natural movement of the viscera. In Avita Yoga, we don't target the viscera directly but let the shapes and resulting freedom of movement in life bring natural movement to these areas.

CHAPTER 13

The Cycle of Healing

Finally, it is time to focus in more detail on healing!

How do we define *healing*? In a way, it's simple: Anything truly healing will interrupt the cycle of pain. Avita Yoga uses shapes to find appropriate entry points into the cycle of pain so that we can begin to undo it. Ideally, the gentle thought of "I want a better way" precedes the shape. Avita teachers are trained to find the favorable entry point in each shape that meets the students *where they are* to allow the undoing to begin. Even if the shape brings instant relief, we may need to use it over time to get closer to the cause. By now, the hidden dangers of simply eliminating pain must be evident—patterns remain, and degeneration can lurk. With gentle willingness, we interrupt the cycle of pain and drop into the healing cycle.

Physiologically, the yoga lights up the parasympathetic nervous system. This leads to the ventral vagal state that increases circulation, digestion, rest, and recuperation.[60] We don't have to study or intellectualize it. We just experience it. We use healing sensation as our barometer. There's nothing to be afraid of in the healing power of *now*. Defensive responses drop, the nervous system calms down, and we react less and respond more. As patterns unwind, we gain trust and take responsibility for our health and mind. Sound healing? It is.

CYCLE OF HEALING

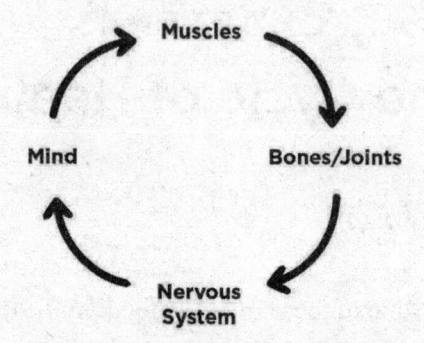

Muscles → Bones/Joints → Nervous System → Mind → Muscles

The moment we repurpose muscles to impact the joints and bones, we gain access to the nervous system, and mind, where all healing originates. Whether active or passive, the Avita shapes, combined with the proper degree of pressure, become the gateway to the formula. Here, in this deep, kind, and powerful moment, we can drop into a peaceful presence from which we observe the healing.

RESOLVING CHRONIC PAIN

When it comes to long-established chronic pain points and patterns, we prefer frequency of practice to intensity of practice. We listen carefully and move slowly so the brain and body can work harmoniously without abrupt sensations triggering a fear response. We let time be on our side.

This section is short because the entire book is dedicated to resolving chronic pain, which always includes a loosening and release of the past, whether tissues, beliefs, or thoughts. By welcoming these sometimes unpleasant feelings and sensations, we use them to show us the way to the light, which is always an inward journey. The way out is in. There is no other way to lasting freedom and joy.

It's not time that heals all wounds. It's repurposing time and using it to unwind and forgive the past. This higher use of time ends our karma and merges us in the healing unity of *now*. The Avita shapes are meant to hasten the inner journey and save you time.

Invite yourself to listen to your body in a new way. Stretch your mind—your thinking—and consider using pain as a "cookie-crumb" trail that takes you to the problem where it can be solved.

HEALING MODE

There is a beautiful shift in perspective as we move away from the concept of fixing to the idea of healing. It's our yoga to use the body, its experiences, and its sensations as a communication device to "move" us into a new perspective on life. It's a way of being. Damage can happen in the body, but in the mind, injury is a choice, not a certainty. And as we salvage our Divine Self, bodily improvements become the evidence that tells us we are moving in the right direction. This is healing mode, and we *want* to get "caught up" in it without attachment to outcome.

We come to the practice to heal because we came into this lifetime to heal. Avita Yoga relies entirely on the will to practice and the feedback it generates. Whether from the body or daily life, it's all about learning to observe, again, *from* a place of peace. This is healing. It is a process of gently taking responsibility not for the problem but for how we see it. We stop pushing the problem onto others. We stop blaming and projecting because all that is given is received. The mind is like a boomerang; giving and receiving are the same. Whatever we try to get rid of comes back, not always felt immediately because it can be hidden and suppressed, only to play out later in a different form.

Let "the buck" stop here. *Now* is a decision we must make. Why delay wholeness and happiness?

INJURY: A HEALING PERSPECTIVE

As with every unwanted event, we often ask, "Why?" Why me? Why did this happen? In a futile effort to figure it out, the ego takes us through a series of hypothetical scenarios. "If only I would have done this or that differently. I should have seen it coming." Yet to ask "why" is accusatory and delays healing. It leads to vicious, fruitless what-if scenarios.

Instead of asking why, ask, "What is this for?" Far more healing than a "positive attitude," asking what any "unwanted" event or diagnosis is *for* is a request to your healed mind for help. It is a way to find and turn the seeming tragedy into a gift. But because injuries and upsets slow us down, the ego will try to solve them quickly to get us back on the same old, well-trodden path. Our ego craves the familiar because it limits and carries past values into the present. Remember, we're here to find a better way, not the former way. If we don't use injuries and mishaps to access the unforgiving thoughts behind them, they are likely to recur in a different form, time, and place.

Let's revisit *Groundhog Day* with Bill Murray. While he didn't break any bones, Phil, the weatherman, was stuck in a harmful, frustrating time loop. Even "death" didn't change it. It's a terrific example of karma and how the same injurious thinking brings recurring problems in different forms. It's our yoga to use every incident, no matter how big or small, to look at the frame of mind *behind* it. The only way Phil could escape the time loop was to honestly examine his perspective and attitude about it. His life became easier and deeply fulfilling as he changed his mind. As he accepted the circumstances around him, he joined and listened to a different inner Voice. He slowed down and found peace within himself.

And there's the gift. True humility is healing because it slows us down and turns us inward. The ego wants to keep racing ahead, doing what we've always done. Keep the status quo no matter the cost. We are given opportunities and situations to slow us down and save time, but do we see them? When I hit one of life's speedbumps do I complain and push on or do I take the hint and slow down a bit? The lesson is often, how can I be truly helpful? We *all* have a healing role, and we are all currently in the perfect situation to lead us to it. Nothing has to change but your perspective. It's our yoga to look deeper and take gentle responsibility for *how* we perceive the world.

There is a hidden gift in every seeming tragedy, and it's our yoga to find it. If we dwell on the problem, we get the problem. But when we use the problem to forgive and accept, the mind opens to what Spirit has in store for us. It will be the road less traveled, and it will be miraculous. There may be injuries, but with this healing frame of mind, you'll soon see there are no accidents.

My first life-changing miracle injury came at the age of twenty-nine: a ski fall that severely hyperflexed my knee. I couldn't walk for a week, so needless to say, I was humbled and forced to slow down. I slowed enough to recognize the invitation to be a model at the first advanced Rolfing training in Boulder, Colorado. The bodywork and insights I received led to a nonsurgical recovery and a career that changed my perspective on yoga. My second miracle injury—the one I described in the Introduction, where Philippe Hartley, pH, and I smashed hips on Vail Mountain—led to the insights and creation of Avita Yoga.

My hip hurt for months after the collision. The impact damaged it, and the trauma irritated the muscles, putting them in spasm, which squeezed the sciatic nerve and sent the pain radiating down the leg. PT, massage, Rolfing, and all the yoga I could muster were not solving the problem. The only way to clean it up was to accept and forgive it with healing shapes and compression. I prayed deeply for a better way, and the answer came through with a massive reorganization of my life and career.

The key was *not* a positive attitude, as many would say. It is the *purpose* given that makes the difference. A positive attitude overrides the trauma and represses grievances. Joining purpose lets the darkness come through where it can be lifted to the light and dissolved. The purpose we *give* life's events is *everything*.

For the most incredible and most purposeful adventure of our lives, we must be willing to give up the specific plans and goals we have for ourselves and follow the intuitive nudges and prompts. It can be unsettling initially, but if we keep trusting and following, it becomes clear that all things work together for good. With the healing power of forgiveness, we can look back and see no accidents, only gifts.

CHAPTER 14
Physical Practice

It's time to bring your body and mind to the practice and get to know them better. Please beware of the tendency to evaluate, whether it's your body, the shape, the class, the pace, or your progress. Do we not move fast enough? Is it too intense? Is it scary? This is your mind coming into the practice and it will find all kinds of reasons to avoid the healing work.

Adjust the pressure for a healing sensation. Allow some space between what you are doing and the mental observation of it. This will make more sense as you practice. It's where healing occurs, and it's why we slow down and listen. Watch the temptation to fidget, adjust clothing, skip steps, breathe loudly, or add variations from other styles—it's all a distraction and ultimately a choice not to drop in, join, and heal.

All Avita Yoga cues are directional. We move one part toward another and stop when the sensation becomes informative. Yogic alignment occurs when the mind is peaceful and confident in the shape with the feedback. This is the meditative part of the practice. We're putting it all together. Watch the tendency to compare and contrast. It's never helpful. There is no competition in a peaceful mind. Find the alignment in heart and mind from within, and good will come.

Here are some guidelines for a successful practice.

1. Eliminate expectations about the shapes. They are potent, and finding a safe entry and sustainable experience in each is essential.
2. Start slow and pace yourself according to the sensation.
3. Don't let the idea that you "can't do yoga" keep you from practicing.
4. If you miss your practice time, it's okay. Don't let the idea of failure keep you from practicing further. Choose again and begin anew.
5. Practice brings results. Remember your goal and use your dedicated time for healing and peace of mind.

WHAT? NO MIRRORS?

Mirrors are meant to inspire and help people find the proper outer alignment, but for what inner gain? Outer reflections can divert us from the inner restrictions, and *samskaras*. If we're not obsessing over our image, we're distracted by someone else's—how they appear and practice. It's inherently competitive, and using the mirror to achieve "proper alignment" may do more harm than good. I've seen plenty of outer alignment that exacerbates an inner problem. If we are constantly concerned about outer appearances, how will we ever look within? How will we unite with Source? If the outer is a representation of the inner, let's work on the inner and let the outer take care of itself.

Which concerns you more, your outer reflection or your inner health? Here's a growth question: "Am I aligned within to the point where there is no inner conflict?" Seem impossible? Only the ego would think so. It wants you to believe the goal of lasting inner peace is unattainable. It does not want you to know the truth and be perfectly happy. But *that* is precisely what you want. Don't be fooled. Dig. Look within and salvage your healed mind.

If yoga means "to join," what am I joining? My reflection? Another body? An ideal physical presentation? No. The physical is not timeless. Yoga is the process and practice of recognizing what has *already* been accomplished, the journey-less journey to Self. It's a path that uses the body to go beyond the body, and it will be delayed if I'm enamored with a reflection.

Practicing in a studio

If you like practicing in person, an internet search may reveal one near you or you may click through to AvitaYogaOnline.com and go to the teacher page. Practicing with a trained Avita Yoga Teacher is a wonderful way to feel cared for and savor the healing container of others in the room sharing the same purpose. Our teachers are in conversation with one another, and we have each other as resources to source the answer for your concerns and questions.

LEVELS OF PRACTICE

Avita is a nonlinear, nonathletic healing approach to yoga that inspires joint health, strong bones, and peace of mind. It works for people of all ages and abilities and relies on time-tested principles consistent throughout all classes.

Avita has three levels: Green, Orange, and Red. They all follow the same safe and sound principles of practice. The magic happens in the Green classes, which is why the vast majority of sequences are Green. Initially, all of my classes were Green, but I found that as pain diminished and mobility increased, students naturally wanted more time, complexity, and pressure. Why? Because they were ready! They recognized and experienced the healing and calming characteristics of compression. I introduced the Orange class once per week, and it became very popular—packed with eighty people in the room—so I added two more and taught three back-to-back for years on Sunday mornings. Eventually I added a limited number of Red classes as yet another option.

Thus, the healing progression of sequences began. Pace yourself and respect the feedback, and, like many beginners, you may enjoy both Green and Orange classes. If it's too much, skip the Orange sequences for a while. I recommend starting with the introductory series 1.0 to understand the concepts of practice.

AVITA YOGA GREEN

The depth and healing happen in the Green classes. They make up most of the practice and require the least amount of effort, which ironically is why people benefit from them. Green classes take a reductionist approach, so neither the body nor the mind is overwhelmed. These classes are all we need in many ways, and people are drawn to their user-friendly nature—a simple way to unwind the complexity of the body. Green Classes are the essential starting place for anyone with injuries, chronic pain, stiffness, or general issues with aging.

AVITA YOGA ORANGE

As mobility and health improve, we naturally desire more time, pressure, and complexity in the shapes and movements. At this point, the student has developed an understanding of Avita and the difference between pain and healing sensation.

Avita Orange classes developed naturally over the years. During the week, I would teach what we later named Green classes, and the popular Sunday classes slowly became more challenging and were dubbed Orange. People loved them, especially those who were more athletically inclined. But people of all abilities enjoyed attending and would often bring visiting family and friends to these classes, even though they were more demanding. Because I was in the room, I could keep my eye on everyone and ensure it was safe and effective.

Nowadays, I'm online, and I follow the same formula: three Green classes followed by one Orange class. Reduce pressure and time if you are ever in doubt. Each series of classes systematically progresses through the body to address all the major joints and bones. Still, skipping the Orange classes is okay until you develop a solid foundation. When ready, you will enjoy the time-tested combination.

AVITA YOGA RED

Few yoga or fitness styles can maintain the same foundational practice goals while increasing intensity. Whether Green, Orange, or Red, we expect the same results—healthy joints, strong bones, and a peaceful mind. This limited series of classes is for those who still believe they need more. It demonstrates that we can have more contemporary shapes and movements and remain focused on health over fitness because we *still* target the joints, bones, and mind.

Lastly, you may enter a search term for classes that target specific body parts and bounce around through the different series. This is okay, but the practice is meant to be a systematic, long-term approach that symphonically works through the body, giving all the parts attention. No two classes are the same, and over one thousand online classes comprise the various series.

FEATURED WORKSHOPS

Having said that, we do offer a more targeted way to get started in Avita using a particular body issue as a starting point. It could be the lower back, hips, shoulders, knees, or neck that leads you to a workshop addressing your ailment. Specific bodily concerns bring many people to Avita. Each workshop covers the targeted area's basic anatomy and guidelines for addressing the problem. It also explains the healing physiology and how it helps cleanse and remodel joints and bones. The workshops include three classes of varying lengths that feature shapes that help restore health and mobility to these specific areas. There's also a downloadable PDF to help you reference the shapes.

Here's the kicker: The shapes you learn in the workshops for your particular concern become "homework." These shapes will bring results, and it's okay to focus on them alone, but the best results come from integrating them as "homework shapes" on off days or after a regular class that may not have had your homework shape in it. Rest days are essential, but the troubled areas need extra attention and practice. It's how I have worked through my knee, hip, and shoulder issues.

PRACTICE MATERIALS

A bolster and a strap are essential items for practice. You may use a firm pillow and a belt as short-term substitutes. Still, in the long run, a 6' yoga strap and a 28" cotton-filled bolster will make practice efficient and enjoyable. The longer bolsters can be found in 10" and 8" diameters. The 10" bolster is the most common and the choice for a medium to large body. The 8" bolster will work for just about anyone, but it is best for a medium or small frame. If in doubt, size up to the 10" bolster.

If the bolster arrives too firm or too big, you can remove a few inches of filling, redistribute, zip it up, and "walk" on it to mash it down. With time they flatten, which is good, but don't buy a rectangular "pre-flattened" bolster. They do not work as well for Avita shapes. To speed up the flattening of cylindrical bolsters and achieve an oblong shape, store your bolster flat with some weight. We prefer cotton filling for the weight and firmness. If you already have one filled with another material like polyester or beans, use it, but when the time is right, invest in yourself and get one filled with cotton.

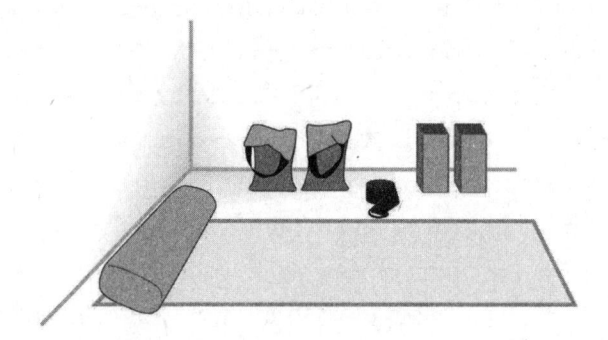

Here's the simple setup: one wall, one mat, one bolster, one strap, two blocks, and two sandbags.

Sandbags ship full or empty. You'll want two. If you order them unfilled, you can buy a bag of play sand at your local hardware store. Use a small scoop and fill it to nine inches. Each inch weighs about a pound, and we aim for nine pounds in each bag. The cotton sandbags that ship empty are much preferred to the material used on most prefilled sandbags. It's more work to buy them empty and fill yourself, but it's worth it. Take them with you to the hardware store; the attendant might help you fill them on the spot. There is no substitute for a cotton sandbag with a strap, but they are the least important and should not delay your practice if you want to get started.

I prefer the lightweight foam blocks. You'll see they are plenty "heavy" for our movements. We use the 3" blocks because they are "grippable" for smaller hands as well as large ones. They are essential in resolving arthritis of the fingers, thumbs, and wrists.

You'll find these material details and sources on the website.

HOW OFTEN? A LITTLE CAN BE A LOT

Do you get distracted and pulled to something "more important" or "more entertaining" than your happiness and health? What pulls you away from meaningful moments with family and friends? What distracts you from being truly helpful? If asked for five minutes of quiet meditation per day, could you do it? Can you repurpose just five minutes out of the 1,440 you have in your day to practice peaceful presence? If it's too painful to sit with your thoughts, that's the reason to do it. Your healed mind wants to be known.

Out of the 168 hours in your week, your bones and joints need only two to four to maintain strength and health. It doesn't take much. Once we plant the seed, a little weeding and nourishment go a long way. As the garden begins to flourish, we enjoy the fruits of our yoga. It's not a matter of readiness but of willingness.

We need enough practice to bring about change, but not so much that it overwhelms the body and mind. Avita is a potent practice, so a little can go a long way. If you practice a few times per week, your entire body will get what it needs through the variety that comes with the progression of classes within each series. If you have particular joint or pain issues, you will have homework shapes to do more frequently. They can be found under featured workshops at AvitaYogaOnline.com.

Can you manage three to four times a week? In the beginning, an *integration* (or rest) day is recommended between practice sessions. We are accustomed to having rest days to give the body time to restore itself, because most forms of exercise involve a catabolic process where tissues are broken down so that they rebuild bigger and stronger. That's not the rationale for Avita Yoga or the rest days.

Avita Yoga cleanses, renews, and restores. The rest days between practice are naturally integrative. The body needs time to integrate the yoga into the nervous system and the millions of cells that make up the various tissues that, in turn, make up the systems that make up the body. The changes need to mesh with daily life. And while we're not tearing anything down to build it back up, we're triggering the body's physiologic mechanisms where cells, tissues, and systems are restored and reorganized to function efficiently.

If your life is hectic and finding time to practice is difficult, watch the tendency to replace frequency with intensity. Try putting your legs up the wall for five minutes a few times a week. This practice should come easy if you follow the inner nudge and let yourself be invited to practice. If you approach it grudgingly or if it feels like work, don't force it.

I imagine a time when Avita Yoga is a regular part of our hygiene for bones, body, and mind. We've conditioned ourselves to brush and floss daily, right? What happens to the teeth and tissues if you don't? Like the bones and joints, we don't feel the pain until too late. With Avita Yoga, you'll benefit from two to three practices a week. Like many students, you may be intuitively drawn to more frequency with time.

HOW MUCH? LESS IS MORE

Asking how much the body can tolerate is a dangerous question. It's better to ask: How much is necessary to heal? It's all about the feedback and peaceful guidance. With a peaceful, confident mind, anything is possible. We practice enough to get results. Why would more be necessary?

"No pain, no gain" is out. Cultivating a meditative practice with heightened kinesthetic and proprioceptive awareness is in. The guided approach to Avita Yoga is a refreshing and simple alternative to exercise. Life has a way of pulling us away from the most meaningful things. It's okay if you miss practice, but don't let guilt reinforce a negative pattern. We all miss practice at times, and it's okay. We pick up where we left off and, with a beginner's mind, meet ourselves in the shape, fresh and new. You never lose your place with Avita. The next class is the right class.

The quest for more keeps us searching and never finding. It keeps inner happiness out of reach by continually dangling carrots in front of us. Inevitably, we realize, just like the country western song suggests, that we're looking for love in all the wrong places. At some point, we recognize the push for more isn't working, and we begin to soften our approach. Eventually, we realize that less is more and that we can relax in timeless peace in all we do.

There is a fitness trend, including many yoga styles, to increase intensity in more imaginative ways. How sustainable and healing is it to flip tractor tires? *More and complex* hides the choice for simple and happy. Physical gains should be a side effect of doing activities we enjoy. The need to "get good" at yoga misses the point entirely. Slowing down for introspection that reveals restrictions and patterns is pushed aside to advance the pose and get it "right." There's no meaning in climbing a mountain *only* to get to the top.

In Avita we ask, "Is it practical?" Will my practice bring me sustainable and practical results? Will it alleviate pain and make my bones and joints stronger and healthier? Will it help me maintain happy function for a lifetime?

"Less is more" is a state of mind, not necessarily a lifestyle. If I gently choose against the ego's need for more or at least notice the fearful desire for more, I move the inner pendulum from scarcity and anxiety to contentment and calm. I don't pursue peace and tranquility; I clear the inner pathway for it to come through naturally.

We know we are advancing when we loosen our attachment to the outcome and find peace with what is. We let the shape do its work while we peacefully observe. When we release thoughts of separation and fear, we automatically advance inward toward joined love.

READY TO GET STARTED?

Now that you have an idea of what getting started looks like, let's turn to the descriptions and shapes that form the foundation of the Avita practice—the subject of the next chapter in our journey together.

CHAPTER 15
Avita Shapes and Movements

Each series includes variations of the shapes in this chapter for a sequential progression through all the joints in your body. Nothing fancy. To experience the foundational principles, equipment, and guidance, visit avitayogaonline.com and watch the three free, introductory videos on Avita basics.

Playlist Series 1.0 corresponds to the shapes described below. It consists of fourteen classes that are between twenty to forty-five minutes long, and will give you a solid understanding of Avita Yoga and likely produce profound results.

The numbered series of sequences are easy to follow as I teach and practice with you. I share my sensations and experiences, making them a relatable and sometimes humorous online experience. My wife says I'm easy to laugh at, but please laugh *with* me too.

Each series consists of thirty-, forty-five, and sixty-minute classes. The first three are Green, and the fourth is Orange. This pattern continues to mimic how I taught in the studio classroom. It's a lovely combination of classes and an excellent starting place for most students. The variation in class lengths makes it easier to fit into your schedule and shows we don't need to overwhelm ourselves to reap the benefits of practice. You'll be amazed at what you can gain with 195 minutes of weekly practice.

Sound like a lot? That's only 3.25 hours per week. If you're like me and many others, you'll find this is a nice schedule to stay healthy and happy. Here we go!

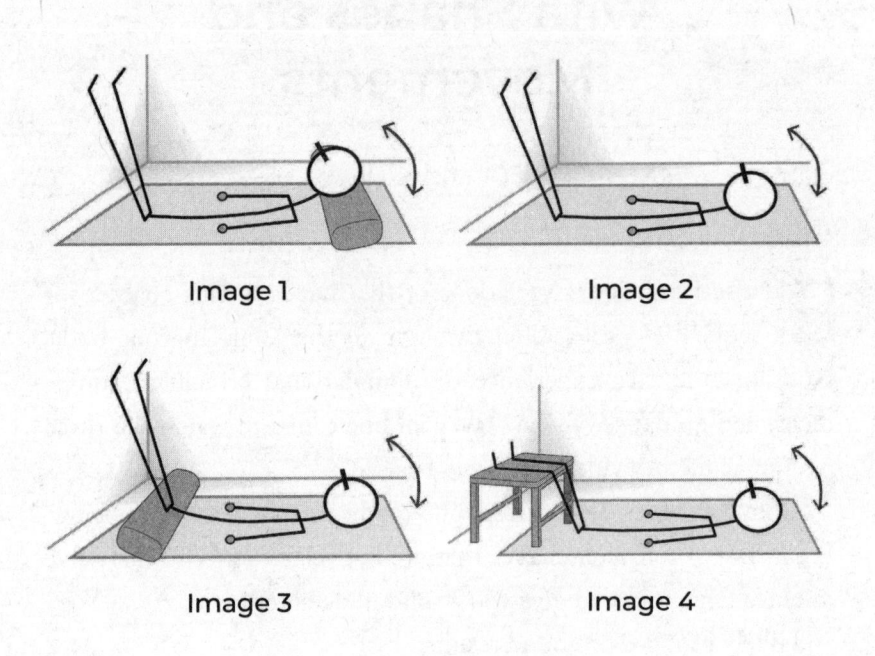

Image 1

Image 2

Image 3

Image 4

VIPARITA KARANI
Legs Up the Wall
Gravity Reversal

There are countless benefits to Legs Up the Wall. It's a relaxing shape we often use to begin a class. Until you decide to prioritize practice, wall space can be hard to find in many households. There is almost always "wall space" in front of a closed door, but you can also benefit by putting your legs over a sofa, ottoman, or chair. This will suffice to relax the lumbar spine, stabilize the sacroiliac joint, reverse the effect of gravity on the body, and provide a remarkable position for many beneficial Avita Yoga shapes. So please do not let the lack of wall space stop you from starting your Avita practice.

Position yourself so the heels can rest on the wall, and the pelvis rests fully on the floor; we want the knees to extend without effort. It's far easier to start closer to the wall and push yourself back than it is to start far away and try to scoot closer to the wall (Image 1).

For ease of entry, make sure your yoga mat is perpendicular to the wall and sit on the edge of the mat with either hip close to the wall. Lie back and roll your legs up the wall simultaneously. You're too close if your knees are bent or your tailbone is off the floor. If this is the case, bend your knees and wiggle back. In a relaxed position, you should feel your sacrum on the floor, the knees extending straight without effort, and the heels on the wall. The feet may turn out to the sides, which is normal. Please note that "straight knees" is a directional cue—perfection is not required. It's okay to feel sensation in the back of the knees, but if it becomes too strong, you may need to start with your legs over an ottoman or chair. Most yoga styles position the sit bones touching the wall, which only works for the very flexible and doesn't allow for the many benefits of using this shape as a sustainable inversion.

Put your bolster crosswise underneath your head and rest your arms at your sides. Slowly turn your head to one side for a profoundly relaxing experience. Many students develop the ability and desire to nap in a shape like this. Passive shapes work while we close our eyes, let go, and relax, which, for an active mind, is easier said than done. For something "to do," observe the sensations in the shape and trust the benefits are far greater than you know. The bolster under the head induces flexion of the cervical spine. It helps resolve tension in the upper back and shoulders, but if you experience neck strain, replace the bolster with a folded blanket or a small cushion.

As you can see from the illustrations, sometimes we rest with the head on the floor (Image 2). However, a thick, muscular upper back or a robust thoracic curve or kyphosis makes it difficult for the head to meet the floor. If so, I recommend supporting your head with a small pillow or soft yoga block.

Numerous movements and variations exist in this shape. Try elevating the pelvis with a bolster or a dense folded blanket. Even a few inches under the pelvis allows the lower back to release toward the floor and relieve any pressure in the pelvis. This alone can help resolve all-too-common pelvic pain (Image 3).

Legs Up the Wall has so many benefits that this shape is the foundation for much of the yoga we do in Avita. In this position, we work with the legs, feet, toes, arms, hands, shoulders, and hips. It's remarkably healing to challenge the body sustainably while in an inverted shape. This is why Avita Yoga is an "endurance activity." We are not running a marathon but deeply challenging the systems, tissues, and cells while encouraging coordinated reorganization among them all.

Imagine the cellular and physiologic reorganization that takes place to endure Legs Up the Wall for twenty to thirty minutes or more. When in doubt, reduce pressure, take a break by bending your knees, or relieve yourself from the shape and wait for the next one. At first, many cannot have their legs on the wall for more than a few minutes. Often, the more athletic cyclists, runners, and weight lifters have a tough time with it because there is so much rigidity in the feet, knees, hips, and lower back. These areas greatly benefit from the Legs Up the Wall position. Again, if the wall is too demanding, start with your legs over a chair or ottoman and work to the wall over time (Image 4). Pace yourself for long-term gains.

Here is a list of potential benefits to Legs Up the Wall:

- It improves circulation to the brain, shoulders, arms, and hands.

- It helps move lymph through the body so it can be cleaned and dumped back into the bloodstream near the heart, which boosts the immune system.
- It helps regulate hormones by taking pressure off the sex organs/glands in men and women.
- It can help resolve pelvic pain and discomfort by encouraging the muscles in the pelvic floor to relax.
- It improves digestion by relaxing the nervous system and taking pressure off the abdomen.
- Elevating the pelvis in this shape reduces pressure on the lower abdominal wall and the inguinal ligament, which can lessen the chances of a hernia.
- It puts a gentle demand on the heart to move the blood up to the toes while not encouraging it to work faster.
- Venous return to the heart, which usually works against gravity, is enhanced and made easy.
- Addresses physical restriction in the ankles, knees, lower back, and neck.
- It helps restore balance to the sacroiliac joints—the lowest part of your spine where the sacrum articulates with the iliac bones of the pelvis.
- It improves mobility of the spine.
- It induces a sense of calm to the body and peace to the mind.
- It relieves symptoms of mild depression and insomnia.
- Along with many other shapes, it restores youthfulness.
- Toxins accumulate at the bottom. This shape reverses the effects of gravity on the feet and legs and helps cleanse and decrease inflammation and swelling.
- It provides an excellent position from which to do a wide range of yoga for the rest of the body and mind.

We often begin and/or end class with this position. Can you see how we maximize the purpose and time in each shape? Never a wasted moment.

AVITA PRACTICE GUIDELINES

1. Remain in the shape 1.5 to 2 minutes
2. Touch into the sensation but don't hunt for it if it's not there
3. Let peace be your guide
4. Discern between pain and healing sensation
5. Reduce time and pressure if necessary

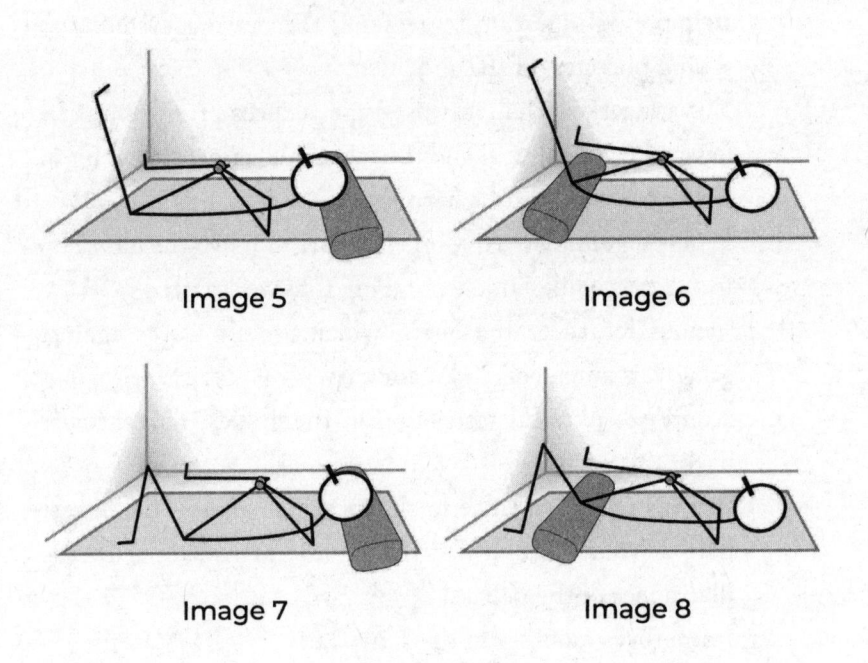

Image 5

Image 6

Image 7

Image 8

APANASANA

Knee to Chest

Hip and Knee Flexion

Bringing the knee to the chest may seem like a simple yoga shape. Yet it is a practical shape that mimics practical movements like washing your feet, putting your pants on, or climbing a ladder. It is a good and straightforward indicator for hip and knee flexion. As you'll see from the images, sometimes we position our legs up the wall, and sometimes with our knees bent and feet on the floor. We interlock the fingers over the knee or behind the knee under the calf muscle. Approach Knee to Chest positions slowly and learn that they are different shapes with different targets. With one focal point or, in this case, one leg at a time, the nervous system is given a single restriction to identify and resolve. While we do introduce complexity at times, we get the best results by addressing the complexities of the body as simply and directly as possible. The mind loves it too. It's like focusing on a single candle flame during meditation. Would it be better to focus on two candles instead of one?

Like any other Avita shape, Knee to Chest should not induce pain. I mention it here because labral tears of the hip are common, and many, believing that pain is gain, will push and make matters worse. Knee to Chest is an excellent shape to slow down and learn what healing sensation is. If you have healthy hips and a flexible constitution, your thigh will be flat on your chest, you won't feel much, and you will want more. More what? Sensation is the guide, *not* the goal. Can you be still and trust the compressive forces are doing their job to keep the knee, hip, and abdominal contents happy and healthy?

To enter the shape, support your head, close your eyes for a peaceful presence, and bring one knee toward the same-side shoulder. Interlock your fingers behind the thigh and let gravity initiate the movement. Slowly apply pressure so that there's a nurturing feeling in the fold of your hip moment by moment. Any stretchy sensation in the back of the thigh should match the compressive feeling in the front of the hip or groin where it's flexing (Image 5). Control the movement to find healing sensation and peace. When in doubt, reduce pressure so you can return and enjoy the yoga another day. Adjust your practice and mind so that time is always on your side.

It's how we reach the bones. Alternatively, elevate the pelvis with a bolster or folded blanket—two or three inches is sufficient to induce lumbar flexion (Image 6).

It's important to vary the support in all the shapes, which is how the sequences are arranged in the online practice. As illustrated, sometimes we support the head (Image 5, 7). At other times, the pelvis is supported, but not the lower back, which induces healthy lumbar flexion. The pelvis should be stable on the bolster as the lower back relaxes toward the floor (Image 6, 8).

Caution: The labrum of the hip is a thin cartilaginous gasket that lines the rim of the socket. It is prone to injury for a variety of reasons. At least one study shows that it is torn in 62 percent of patients over fifty years.[61]

If torn, it will likely present with pain in the groin that feels like a muscle strain. If you feel deep organic pain in the groin or fold of the hip, you may have a torn labrum. Fear not, many lead happy and productive lives with this condition, but continually pressing on it will only make it worse. You may safely explore the shape described above but stay out of the pain.

There are two key measures for shoulder health: the possibility of interlocking the fingers under the head, and the movement potential of reaching fully overhead with elbows straight. Neither movement is taken for granted, and many Avita students gently work with one or the other to improve joint health. We will cover these two shapes next.

Image 9

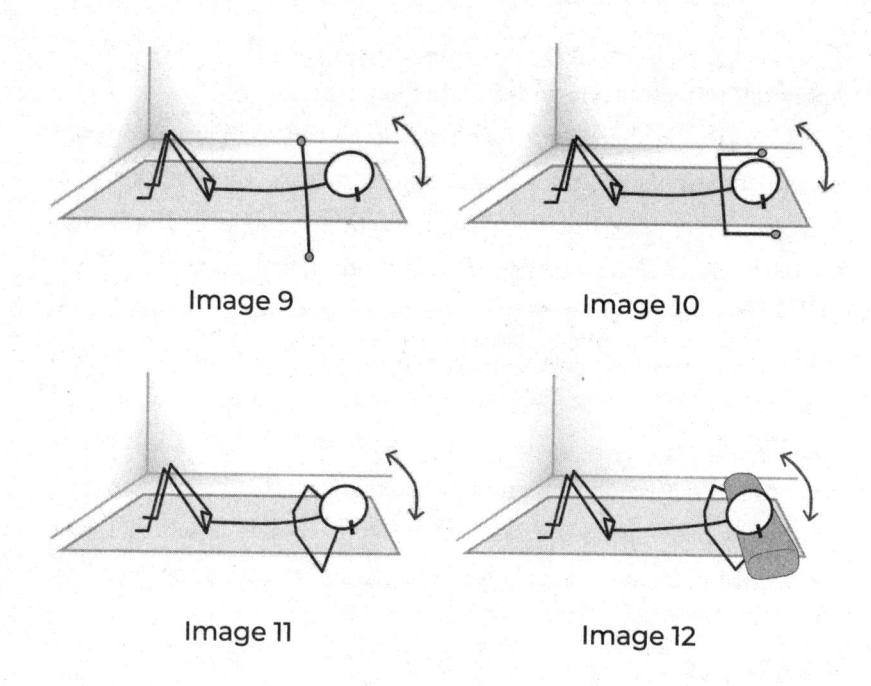

Image 10

Image 11

Image 12

SUPTA ANUVITTASANA
Interlocking Fingers Behind the Head
Practical Shoulder Mobility

Here, we are moving the arms toward full flexion and external rotation. Consider this shape a fundamental precursor to washing your hair or putting on a T-shirt. Every shape and movement must make practical sense.

While we move toward the "ideal," it is never the goal. What is the goal? *Peace.* Class by class, we address the restrictions that show up without evaluation or judgment. Most can begin with the arms out to the sides in a T shape (Image 9). From there, we bend the elbows toward 90° to goal-post arms (Image 10). We move toward interlocking the fingers under the head (Image 11) and eventually under the bolster (Image 12). For many, interlocking the fingers under the bolster like this takes time and practice, but that's what time and practice are for. Touching into the healing sensation and spending peaceful time with it is the key.

Change the shape or reduce pressure if you feel nerve pain, tingling, or numbness. It's not uncommon to take short naps or fall asleep in shapes like this and wake up with a numb arm. That's not a cause for alarm. Keep the peace in your mind, and gently release the shape, moving slowly, noticing the change in sensation in your arms and hands. Something is causing the restriction on either the flow of blood or the nerves. We stand the best chance of resolving it by moving slowly, touching into the limitation at the point just before the onset of nerve-tingling, numbness, or pain. There is no gain with pain or by listening to the voice of fear and avoiding practice. Take a kind and consistent approach, and let time and gravity be on your side.

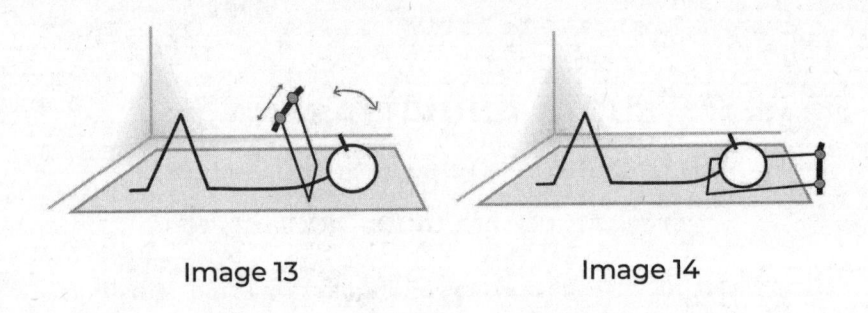

Image 13

Image 14

SUPTA HASTASANA

Overhead Reach

Practical Shoulder Mobility

One of the most valuable and practical indicators of shoulder health is our ability to reach overhead. Why? Reaching overhead expresses a full range of motion; full function means the joint is healthy. But we cannot skip steps. Joints and bones heal *as* we move them toward their full potential. This is radically different than simply advancing the movement for a greater range of motion.

The problem begins when we stop using the full expression of movement. Do you remember hanging from monkey bars when you were a kid? It was good for your shoulders. Not only do we not hang from our hands and climb trees anymore, but we're conditioned to stop the movement when it's painful, or we can no longer "do it." To work *with* the fear and pain, we start on the floor where we don't have to fight gravity. We mimic hanging from our hands, which is incredibly healing for the shoulders, elbows, wrists, hands, and fingers.

Again, overhead reach is the first movement we lose because we stop doing it. Funny enough, hand-to-mouth is the last movement to go. This is a prime example of the universal "use it or lose it" theory. What reason do you have to extend your arms overhead fully? Even pressing weights overhead is insufficient because loaded and repetitious movement will not heal and remodel the joint—and could damage it further. We need prolonged compression with a calm mind to bring the restoration. Sure, hanging from monkey bars has stretchy qualities in some areas. But do not underestimate the value of the compressive forces occurring in the bones of the fingers, hands, elbows, and shoulders when hanging. Generally, we use shapes like this to regain the ability to hang from our hands sustainably. Whether we attain that possibility matters not.

Shoulder restrictions are exposed and resolved with elbow extension while moving the arms overhead and toward the body's center line. Regardless of the body part, we meet the restriction where it is and watch helpful changes occur class by class.

First, lie on your back with your knees bent and your feet flat on the floor. Find a yoga strap or belt and fold it in half, usually twice, so you don't have tails dragging along the floor. Extend your arms toward the ceiling, with hands over your shoulders, and tug on the strap as if to stretch it between your hands. Close your eyes and feel. Straighten your elbows. Keep the details, pressing toward the ceiling with the arms perpendicular to the floor and the fingers gripping evenly (Image 13).

Slowly lower your arms overhead toward the floor, reaching for the wall behind you (Image 14). Go very slow because, more than likely, you will be moving into shoulder irritation or impingement. Can you stay serene as you move with all the details, squeezing the fingers, putting traction on the strap between your two hands, and extending the elbows while simultaneously touching into the impinged area? This is the yoga. This is what brings healing to the shoulder and restores the movement.

After one to two minutes, diminish the effort and go even slower on the return, raising your arms back toward the ceiling. Let the shoulders sink down into the floor as you raise the arms up. When complete, rest your arms at your sides, palms up.

This shape has many variations because the shoulder moves in infinite ways, and as I say in class, we want to contact them "all." As we find our way into the restrictions and resolve them, the overhead reach is restored. Increasing the range of motion without healing along the way is a mistake. Why? Because it's much more challenging to go back and catch the arthritis and degeneration if you have skipped the steps. Working with the resistance is the key to resolving it.

The overhead reach is one of the most healing things we can do for the shoulders, but we do it slowly and confidently, so we mend along the way. Regardless of the joint, if you have full range of motion and don't use it, it will degrade, and you'll eventually lose it. Whether it becomes painful or not is a different story. Whether lying down or standing, the healthy movement potential for the shoulders is hands together, above and slightly behind the head, with both elbows straight. If you have it, why not keep it? Working toward it keeps the arms and shoulders healthy regardless of the range of motion.

This movement promotes lymphatic drainage around the armpits and can help diminish puffiness in this area. It's an early indicator that your lymphatic system needs attention. Swollen lymph nodes may be a sign of infection, a lack of movement, or illness.[62] I have had breast cancer survivors in my classes who used this shape and movement to regain mobility after surgery. This area becomes delicate because connective tissue and lymph nodes are removed. Scar tissue is essentially disorganized fascia produced to mend anything the body perceives as traumatic or invasive. These sustained movements help resorb and remodel these tissues to promote lymphatic and blood flow, reduce the build-up of scar tissue, restore health, and, lastly, increase range of motion.

Image 15

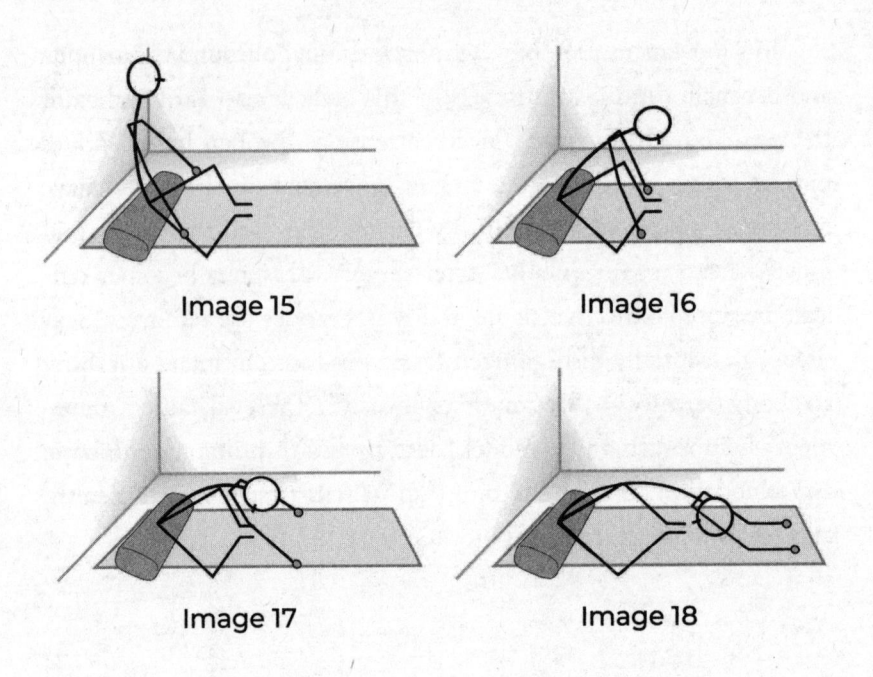

Image 16

Image 17

Image 18

BADDHA KONASANA

Flexion and External Rotation of Hips

Lower Back Flexion

Place your bolster horizontally to the wall and a palm width away. Sit on it so you feel your sit bones centered front and back on the bolster and bring the soles of your feet together. Rest against the wall and move your heels out 12" to 18". Close your eyes and observe (Image 15).

Slowly curve forward. Keep your shoulders, arms, and hands relaxed at your sides shoulder-width apart or more. Use your hands against the floor to prevent the sensation from becoming too strong in the hips or lower back as you curve (Image 16, 17, 18).

With your lower legs forming a diamond shape the legs act as a cantilever, encouraging your entire spine to curve. We aim to feel the rigidity in the hips *and* lower back, the targeted areas for the shape. With time and practice, the knees will drop toward the floor, signifying the hips' release, while the lower back releases and gains flexion. Do not try to advance the shape by pulling on your feet, and resist bringing your feet in close to the bolster because you will lose the leverage needed to encourage lumbar flexion.

If your hips are looser than the lower back, the knees will drop, and the lower back won't curve as you bend forward. This means most of the forward flexion comes from the hips, not the lower back. In this case, there is a tendency to slide off the bolster onto the floor. If this is happening to you, press your feet into the floor, keep the sit bones centered on the bolster, and isolate the stiffness in the lower back. It will take a unique effort to do this, but with kind, consistent practice, the hips will develop stability, and the lower back will start to move. Many accomplished yogis and dancers have loose hips and a stiff lower back. Because of their conditioning, they may resist this atypical approach to Baddha Konasana, which isolates and mobilizes the stiffness in the lower back. Remember, we want small, incremental changes over time and practice.

I often refer to the lower back as the dark side of the moon. We can't see it, and we cannot feel the lack of movement in the lumbar region because the hips will compensate for it. People can have lower back pain but don't usually feel lower back stiffness. We don't think it's a problem until years down the road when the lack of movement in the lumbar vertebrae calcifies and infringes on the spinal cord. Surgery for this condition, called stenosis, is usually quite successful. The yoga is for those who catch the problem soon enough and prefer to avoid surgery.

Image 19

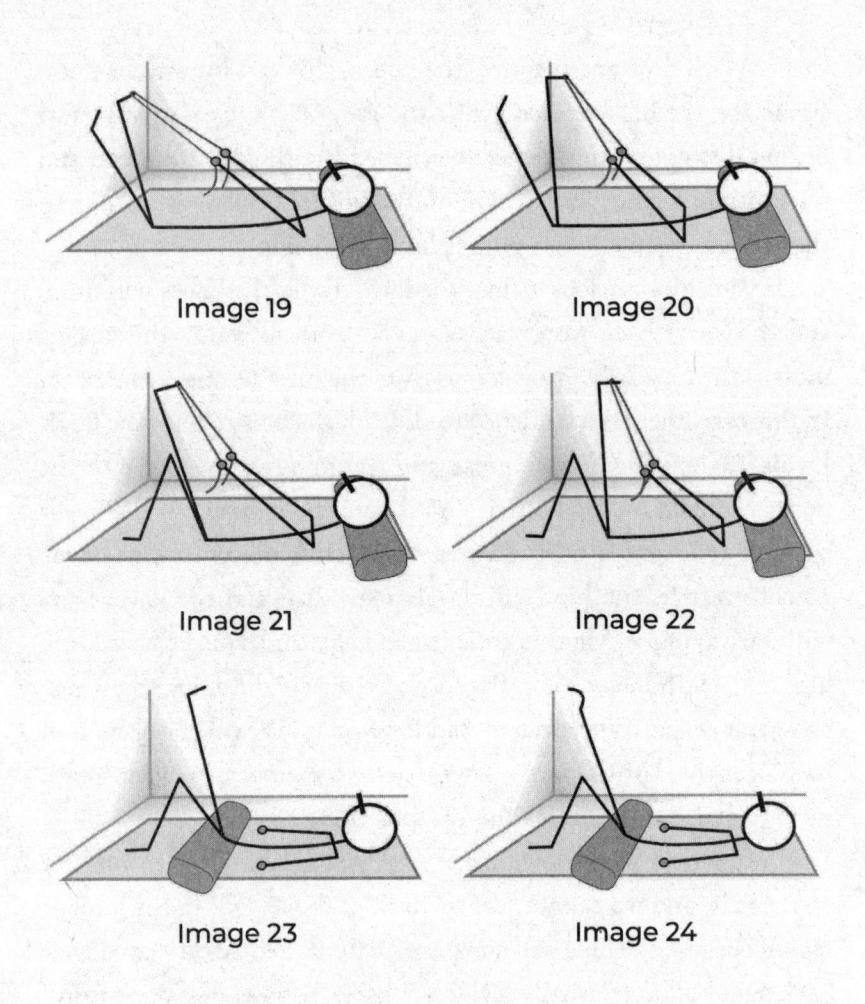

Image 20

Image 21

Image 22

Image 23

Image 24

SUPTA PADANGUSTASANA

Knee Extension with Strap Work

Most people will look at these figures and assume the shape is meant to stretch the hamstrings. I've yet to see a new student not take this approach and launch into a hamstring stretch. Conventional yogic thinking is almost always about advancing the shape and stretching something. Why would you put the strap around your foot if it were not meant to stretch the hamstrings?

Here's why. In Avita Yoga, we use this position to improve the joint health of the fingers, hands, shoulders, toes, ankles, and knees. The muscles become strong and supple because we use them to strengthen and condition bones and joints. We use the strap to support the shape to get into the foot, leg, and hip bones. As you'll see in the illustrations, sometimes we have the same shape without the strap. As long as the soft tissues are ready, the passive shapes take us inward, closer to the bones. When muscles activate, they tug on the bones and squeeze them in multiple directions. This won't make sense until you try some of the shapes and feel your way into the Avita approach. Remember, we use the active shapes to "earn" our way into the passive ones.

One leg at a time, start with the knees bent and the feet flat on the floor. Put the strap around the ball of one foot and extend the knee so both knees are the same height (Image 21). The idea is to have the height or angle of your leg low enough to extend the knee with minimal effort. The strap's purpose is to help support the leg in this position. You may feel a restriction in the upper calf and the back of the knee, and you will be inclined to protect this area and go for a hamstring stretch. Diminish pressure and use the wall if necessary. The strap is too much for some, and we initially resort to holding the shape without it. It's work, and often, the muscled athletes have the most restriction in the back of the knee. When do they extend it fully, running, riding a bike, or playing tennis? There may be a "stretchy" feeling in the back of the knee, but compressive forces are occurring in the front behind the patella. Flexion of any joint, in this case the knee, will benefit by working on extension, and vice versa. Don't get stuck going in one direction. If you want more flexion of the knee, work on extension too. Regardless of the joint, flexion aids extension, and extension aids with flexion.

Further, when we engage one set of muscles, like the quadriceps, to straighten the knee, the antagonistic muscles, like the hamstrings and calf muscles, are asked to release, not to stretch! It's called reciprocal inhibition, and we rely on this fundamental principle in every shape we enjoy. It's in the physiology books, but we don't read it closely enough.

Note the position of the hands on the strap. Most beginning students wrap the strap around their hands, bend their elbows, and pull their leg closer to them, mainly to avoid the more profound yoga. There is a better and more helpful approach, but it will take willingness initially. Keep your hands high and avoid the temptation to wrap the strap around your hands. Instead, rely on the musculature in your fingers and thumbs to hold the strap with the elbows reasonably straight (Images 19-22). This allows the shoulders to relax away from the ears and drop toward the floor. Sustaining the shape alone takes effort because we are not accustomed to using our fingers and hands while relaxing the shoulders. This is a massive release that will come with time and practice. In the short term, wrapping the strap around your hands for a brief respite is okay. Like any Avita shape, it gets easier as restrictions are resolved and systems are reorganized.

We usually hold the shape for one to two minutes with the eyes closed, breathing in and out of the nose. Sometimes I cue to bring the leg closer (Images 20, 22), but not at the cost of bending the knee, where the restriction is often found. We practice fully extending the knee and contacting the restriction, scar tissue, trauma, and compensatory patterns that limit the extension of the knee. Variations with plantar flexion (Image 24) and dorsiflexion (Image 23) of the foot come with different placements of the strap on the arch, heel, and ball of the foot, or with no strap at all, as illustrated.

Those with a flexible constitution are deeply attracted to the stretch sensation in the musculature and will attempt to bring the leg past vertical. But doing so has no benefits and comes with risk. Elongated hamstrings can lead to destabilization of the knee and lower back. Go for the bones and find the healing sensation in and near the knee. The stretchy feeling is fine; it's just not the goal.

Image 25

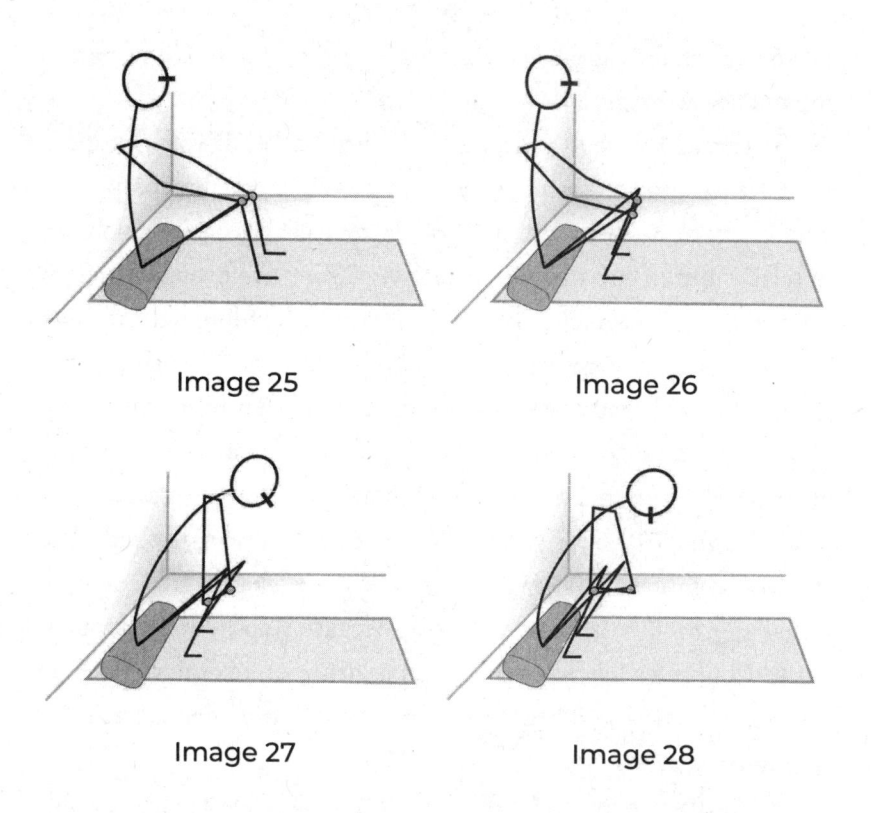

Image 26

Image 27

Image 28

MALASANA

The Long-Lost Squat

Full Body Flexion and Compression

When was the last time you squatted on the floor? We see children and kids do it all the time. When did we stop the squat? Years ago, squatting was a requirement to either relieve ourselves in the woods, forage, or sit around the fire. When I traveled through Africa in the 1980s, I noticed how people waiting for the bus were often in Malasana. While serving in a medical clinic in Nepal, I noticed people waiting their turn sitting in Malasana. If you have ever used a squatty potty in a Third World country you understand the value of having a good squat. I sometimes joke that creature comforts of toilets and chairs have caused more harm than good. Convenience comes at what cost?

Squatting is a good measure of physical health. If you can squat, you have foot and ankle mobility, and your knees can flex completely. Your hip flexion is complete, and your lower back has enough mobility to release into a curve, while your lower front has enough space to welcome the movement. It's healing for the abdominal contents because it brings compression onto the intestines, liver, and other vital organs. All body parts love compression. They're stimulated by it. They're massaged and encouraged to move and slide against each other by it, not to mention it's a profoundly relaxing position.

Have you lost your squat? Find it, but not by trying to squat. The shape we might want is *not* the one that will develop it. This compromised approach will come with costs because steps will be skipped. Instead, consider the many Avita shapes designed to remove the barriers to a practical and healthy squat. Practice, and what is meant to be will come naturally.

Begin by placing the bolster a few inches away from the wall, have a seat on it, and rest your hands on your knees (Image 25). This alone can bring plenty of feedback for those who have not squatted in a while. If this is true for you, come to this version of the shape frequently and continue working through a series of classes to resolve hip, lower back, knee, and ankle rigidity. With time and practice, you will be able to bring the heels closer to the bolster and maintain a curved spine (Images 26, 27, 28). Don't force it, and be weary of deep organic pain that can be indicative of a torn labrum, as described earlier, when bringing the knee to the chest. It's the same movement, with potentially more pressure. It's safe, just listen carefully. Everything we do in Avita Yoga can lead you toward a healthy squat and walk.

Image 29

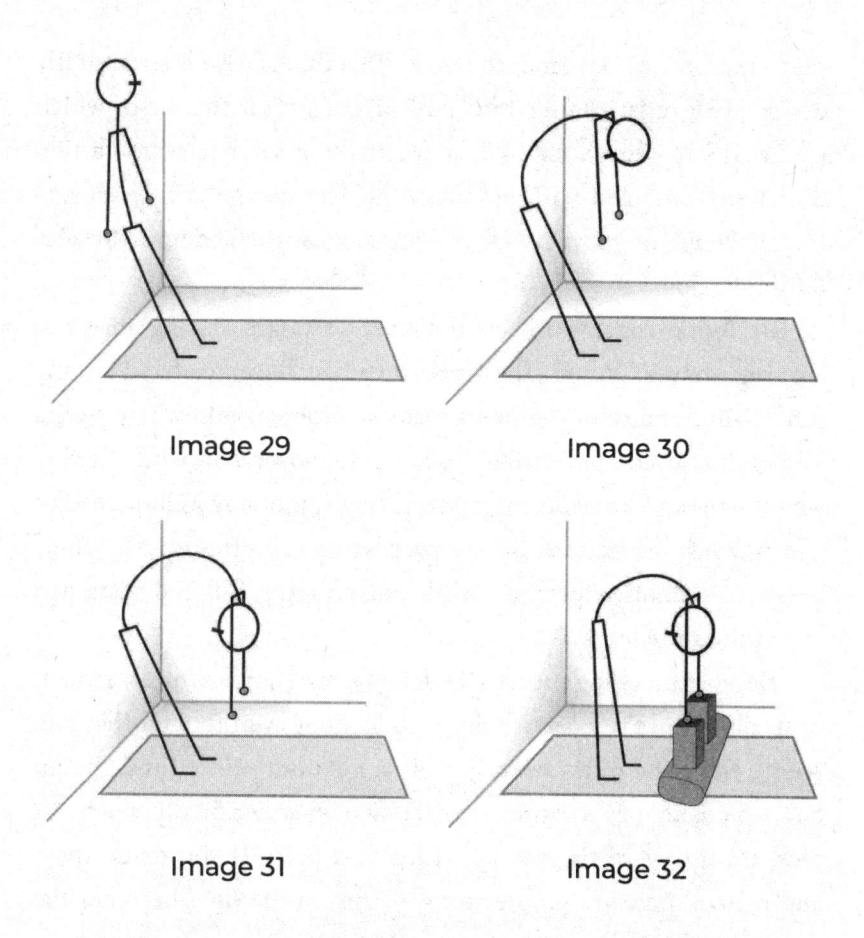

Image 30

Image 31

Image 32

UTTANASANA

Standing Forward Curve

Knee Extension and Spinal Flexion

In Avita Yoga, whether standing or seated, the forward curve is always about mobilizing the lower back and inducing congruent spinal flexion. These articulations are vulnerable because they have been overly protected, so we target them very slowly and kindly. The illustrations (Images 29, 30, 31) exaggerate the potential for most, so don't be aggressive and try to make yourself look like the stick figure. We underestimate the importance and difficulty of lumbar flexion because of the thick thoracolumbar fascia and muscle layers that support the body from the back. This thick fascia is structurally designed to resist the forward pull of gravity on the torso, which means it can also work against us, making vital forward flexion difficult. Combined with any desire to harden the abs, it adds to the challenge of getting vital compression in the abdominal cavity during flexion.

In Avita Yoga, we keep the knees straight during forward, curving shapes. Why? The knees need to be extended like any other joint, and doing so helps identify problems elsewhere. Avita Yoga is a non-compromising approach to movement, which is why we go slow and leave nothing out. Extension of any joint identifies and releases restrictions in one part while bringing healthy compression to another part, all while encouraging full and sustained use of the muscles.

Because touching the toes has long been a standard measurement of flexibility, we've been conditioned to do it even though they can seem a thousand miles away. We either get disappointed and give up or keep pushing as if salvation will dawn when we finally touch our toes, regardless of the compensation and pain. If you touch them and realize there are no fireworks, palms on the floor becomes the next goal. Forget about it!

The forward curve is a function of many moving parts, including the extension of the knee, a release in the Achilles tendon, calf muscles, connective tissue, and the foot's plantar fascia. We use the shape to improve the spine's ability to flex with the hips for practical everyday movement. Yes, the hamstrings must extend for this movement to happen, and while they are blamed for the limit on the shape, they are not the problem. They are merely doing their job of stabilizing the pelvis so the lower back can flex and move in various ways.

To begin, walk your feet 16" to 20" away from the wall and lean against it. It should feel like you're relying on the friction underneath your feet and the wall for support. Allow your arms to hang at your sides and keep them relaxed throughout the movement. Draw the belly in while moving your tailbone down, sit bones toward your heels, and lumbar spine toward the wall. Maintain for about a minute while refining the shape and relaxing your arms at your sides (Image 29).

Keep your legs engaged and knees straight, and slowly curve forward without straining your head and neck or reaching with your arms and shoulders. Engaging the legs while relaxing these other parts takes focus, so stop periodically to verify. Have no agenda about touching your toes or advancing the shape. Instead, keep refining, firming the thighs, and moving the tailbone down. What group of muscles keeps the tailbone from sliding up the wall? The hamstrings. Engage them. It won't be easy to feel them working, but keeping the tailbone moving down will activate them. Lift the abdominal muscles to help curve your spine (Images 30, 31).

Abs up, belly up, tailbone down. Don't reach with your arms, head, neck, or shoulders; instead, allow them all to hang. Reaching forward in these shapes only adds to typical patterns and movements like an exaggerated thoracic curve and forward head posture. Do you feel stiffness in your lower back? Yes or no, it matters not.

At some point, the tailbone may start to slide up the wall. It's okay to relax and hang in the shape *if* you feel safe and confident on all levels. After about thirty seconds, firm your thighs, lead with the tailbone, move it down the wall, lift the abs, and slowly reverse the process, paying close attention to your relaxed arms, shoulders, neck, and head. The idea is to lift with the abs and raise yourself by drawing the sit bones toward the heels, utilizing hamstring muscle engagement.

Once up, firm your lower back to the wall and relax the upper body as we did when we started. Close your eyes, and let the floor and wall support you briefly before stepping back and taking a short walk.

When not using the wall, we often provide support for the hands to help support the shape and keep a consistent focus on the total curvature of the spine. Depending on one's flexibility, support for the hands may be added or removed (Image 32). Touching the floor with the knees straight is no indication of healthy spinal movement. Many have been conditioned to "hinge at the hips" and "swan dive" into a forward fold, which targets the hamstrings. There is often a cue to "micro-bend" the knees, isolating and supporting knee restrictions and limiting active use of the ligaments within the knee. Even the meniscus wants compression and consistent use to stay healthy. We thoughtfully use the quadriceps to extend the knees to condition them inside and out.

Remember, use it or lose it. But if it's been a while since you have actively used the ligaments in your knees, go slow and approach the shape with ample support, even if it's easy to touch your toes. The supine strap work illustrated earlier puts us in a safer and more controlled relationship with gravity, which prepares the body and mind for standing shapes like this.

Image 33

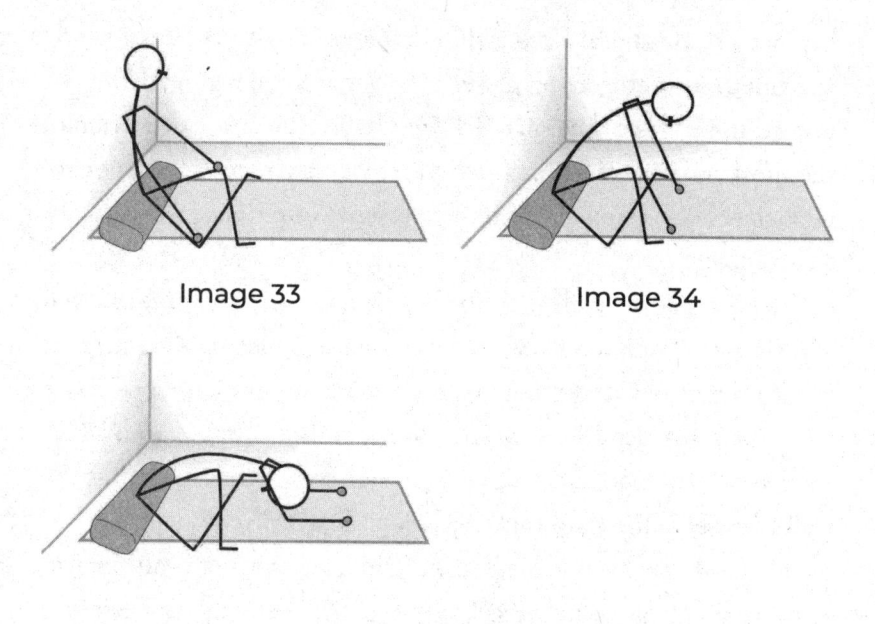

Image 34

Image 35

SUKHASANA

Sitting Legs Crossed

External Rotation of the Hips and Flexion of the Lumbar Spine

We get more mileage out of Sukhasana than just about any other shape. Why? Because "easy pose," approached through the eyes of Avita Yoga, takes the hips into vital external rotation and simultaneously brings flexion to the hips and lower back. We often see Sukhasana demonstrated with the heels drawn in close, sometimes with the feet stacked on each other because it's comfortable and avoids the deeper restrictions. Resist the desire to pull the heels close to the groin for comfort. You won't get the results.

In Avita Yoga, we move the feet away from the bolster so that the lower leg closest to you is parallel to the end of the mat. The leg farthest away will have a slightly bigger angle. We then subtly attempt to move the knees closer together and the feet farther apart toward the edges of the mat. This results in a clear identification of the most prominent hip restriction. If we catch this soon enough, it can be cleaned up, and from my personal experience, surgery can be avoided.

We start at the wall with the bolster a few inches from the wall and sit bones centered front and back, with one leg crossed in front of the other. Look down and make the adjustments mentioned above with the closest leg to you parallel to the wall in front of you. Move your feet to the sides a bit, then close your eyes and relax against the wall to observe the shape and sensation (Image 33).

What do you feel? Does it bring up a memory of a hip injury? Are you able to genuinely relax in the shape? At times, stiffness and restriction are so strong that little to no sensation is felt. Gravity is not enough in these situations, so we sometimes apply sandbags to the thighs to bring the necessary pressure and move into the restricted territory. Sensation is the guide. Too strong, reduce pressure. Never do we add weight to advance the shape alone. Advances in the shape should always come as pleasant surprises.

Slowly curve forward, eyes closed, observing the shape from the inside. What do you feel as you curve forward? With your neck and head relaxed, let the shoulders be easy, and have your elbows slightly bent and hands at your sides (Image 34). Be willing to bump into the restriction and spend some time with it; don't let the sensation be intense in the soft tissues, outer hip muscles, and hamstrings. If you feel strong feedback in these areas, it's likely because of a hip restriction being felt in the soft tissues. In this case, diminish pressure by raising yourself some and supporting with your hands more. The "closer" you are to the bones and joints, the safer it is. Image 35 illustrates the full potential of the shape. There is never a need to go for a certain look. Avita Yoga is an inside job.

After one to two minutes, slowly raise, rest against the wall, switch the cross of your legs, and pause. Open your eyes and check to see that the shin closest to you is parallel to the wall in front of you. Move your feet laterally a bit and slowly curve forward. If the sensation stays strong in one hip, regardless of which leg is in front, it can indicate an issue in that particular hip. Of course, both hips could have issues, but that's rare because compensatory patterns are usually not bilateral. If the sensation is relatively equal side to side, it could mean your hips are in pretty good health. Please work with the feedback and resist the desire to evaluate. Observe your thoughts and feelings forgivingly, adjust the pressure by raising if needed, and be in the moment. After one to two minutes, raise yourself and rest against the wall without changing the shape. As in any shape, pause before reacting and trying to eliminate sensation unless cued otherwise. Get in touch with the quick need to react versus the gentle ability to respond. We don't want to interfere with the healing physiology.

Sometimes we move into a new shape at this point, but for now, please stand up and walk. Don't be surprised if standing up is challenging, and don't be surprised if you walk with a limp. Walk *through* the limp until you achieve a regular walk. Congratulations! You just completed your first Sukhasana, and there will be more like it and many variations that will have healing benefits for your hips. Your walk will get better and better.

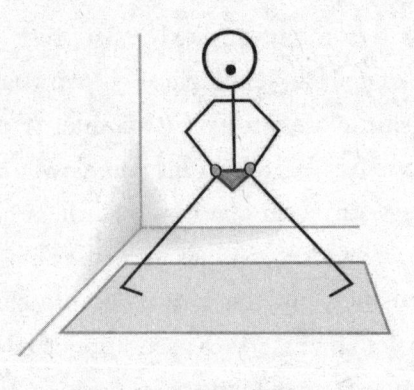

Image 36

PRASARITA PADDOTANASANA
Standing, Legs Wide
Internal Rotation of Hips

This is the counterpose to Sukhasana. The knees are straight, and the hips are internally rotated. Between these two shapes, Sukhasana and Prasarita Paddotanasana, the hips undergo an extensive range of movement. We rarely use Sanskrit terminology because it's much more helpful to explain the way in and out of the shape, the benefits, and the possible sensations. However, naming it in Sanskrit can sometimes offer a quicker reference than describing it in English.

Here's the way in. Standing with your legs wide, align the heels with the back edge of the mat and turn them out. The toes point in as a result of the heels out. The stance is broad but not so wide that you can't effectively straighten the knees and turn the tailbone down toward the floor. Remember, there's no one to impress. We're simply exposing restrictions primarily through knee extension and internal hip rotation.

Engage the gluteal muscles and hamstrings to move the tailbone toward the floor and the pubic bone toward your nose. This movement engages the musculature, adding compression throughout the hip joints, encouraging lumbar flexion, and increasing compressions through the knees down into the feet and ankles. We maintain for about a minute.

This is the baseline for many standing shapes, including warrior and triangle variations. We also do arm, shoulder, and knee work in this shape, which will come through the online or classroom sequences. It's a relatively simple shape with many benefits that require nothing more than a little willingness.

Image 37

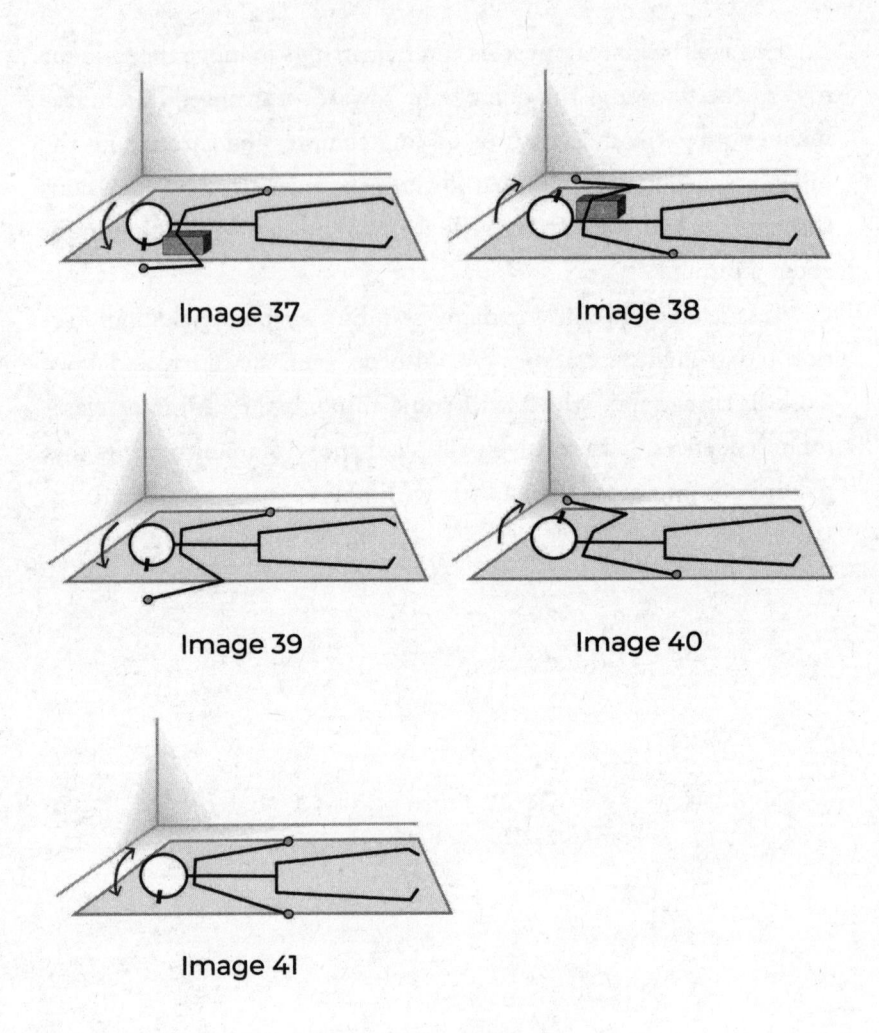

Image 38

Image 39

Image 40

Image 41

SHITHILASANA

Tummy Time

Neck Mobility

Tummy time is not just for infants. Yes, time on the tummy is vital for little ones, especially in early development. It compresses the body's front side during unprecedented cellular division and growth. And it's not just about bones, joints, and muscles. Tummy time and other resting positions stimulate nerve growth through compression, gravity, and pressure, which is why there is a thing called infant massage.

We can recapture the benefits of tummy time as adults. It can be an incredibly challenging shape if the neck is rigid, which, more often than not, makes the neck the target of the shape. Give it a try and see if you can lie on your belly with the toes turned in, and the heels turned out. Place your hands back by your sides, palms up. Turn your head to one side to rest with your eyes closed, and observe the compressive forces (Image 41).

If it's too demanding on your neck, support the shoulder on the side to which your head is turned. There are a few ways to do this. One is to bring your hand up by your face (Image 39, 40). If you need more support, try placing a blanket or a soft yoga block under your shoulder (Image 37, 38). Lifting this part of your torso should diminish the pressure on the neck so you can rest peacefully. After one to two minutes, lift your head and gently turn to the other side, knowing that you may have an entirely different experience in the other direction. It may or may not need the same support as the previous side. Use necessary support to make this a relaxing position with mild sensation. With time and practice, you can lessen the support as resolutions come. In Avita we allow the simplicity of the shape to work on the complexity of the body.

Image 42

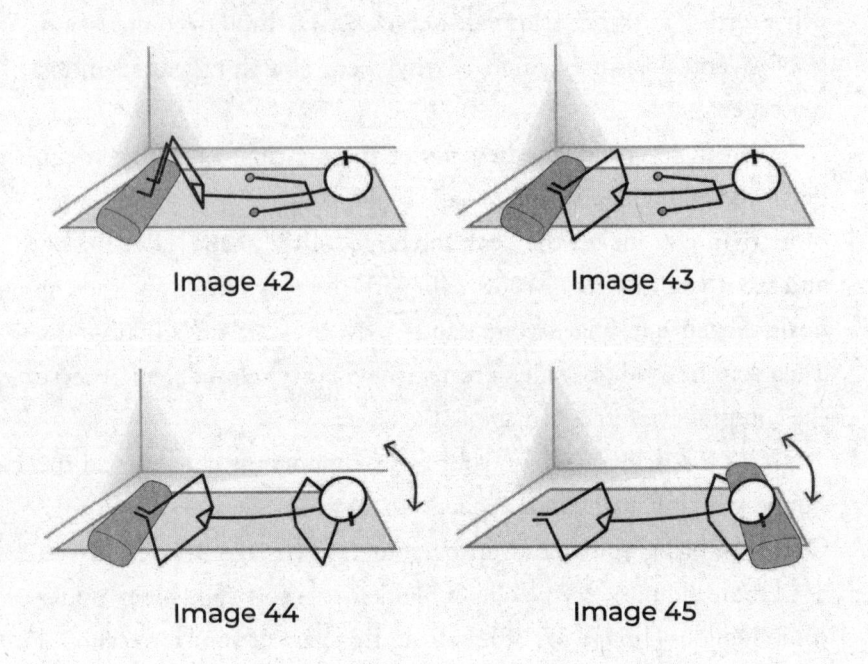

Image 43

Image 44

Image 45

SUPTA BADDHA KONASANA
Reclined External Rotation of the Hips
Hip and Shoulder Mobility

Lie on your back with your knees bent and your feet flat on the bolster. Be sure the bolster position feels supportive. If it's too far away, the lower back will move away from the floor, and if it's too close, it won't feel relaxing. Have your arms at your sides (Image 42).

Bring the soles of the feet together, allowing the knees to slowly drop laterally toward the floor (Image 43). What do you feel? Moving according to the feedback, you may need to use the inner thigh muscles to hold the knees up so the sensation is not too strong in the groin or hip. The sensation of stiffness can show up in the inside medial part of the hip and thigh, while a cramping or pinching sensation can sometimes be felt in the outer hip. If you're moving thoughtfully and slowly, you can sustain the shape peacefully and let it work *for* you. As restrictions resolve with time and practice, the knees will drop, and you may maintain the shape passively and peacefully for one to two minutes.

Unlike many forms of yoga, we rarely use blocks and props to support and make the shape more comfortable. Why? We cannot protect our way into better health. Supporting the shape protects the restriction and problematic patterns. It's *not* our yoga to seek comfort; it's our yoga to find and remove the barriers to it. This is why we take an active, thoughtful approach to every shape until we can enjoy it passively. Use the inner thigh muscles to hold the knees up to manage the sensation in the shape properly. Keep the knees the same height so the back of the pelvis is balanced evenly on the floor.

Avita Yoga has many shapes on the floor that often mimic the body when standing. We put ourselves in friendly relationships with gravity so that it works for us, not against. It allows us to spend the needed time in the shapes, without excessive effort, which is needed for change to occur. We need a simple way to access the complex nature of the body and mind and all its "doings." We cannot solve a complex, multilayered pattern with a complex and demanding approach. Why struggle with the tree pose when you could lie on your back and work on both hips simultaneously in Supta Baddha Konasana? Granted, every shape has unique benefits, but it's too easy to fall into inner competition with yourself and try to perfect the "pose." Why fight with the triangle pose, which requires external rotation of the hips, and risk tweaking your SI joint, when you could spend productive time addressing the hips in a relaxed manner on the floor?

This shape has many variations, all of which can have active and passive qualities. We put the bolster in various positions to expose restrictions and encourage vital spine and hip movement. As shown, I often add neck turns and shoulder work to the shapes (Images 44, 45.) But don't add complexity too quickly. If we overwhelm the nervous system, results will be delayed.

Image 46

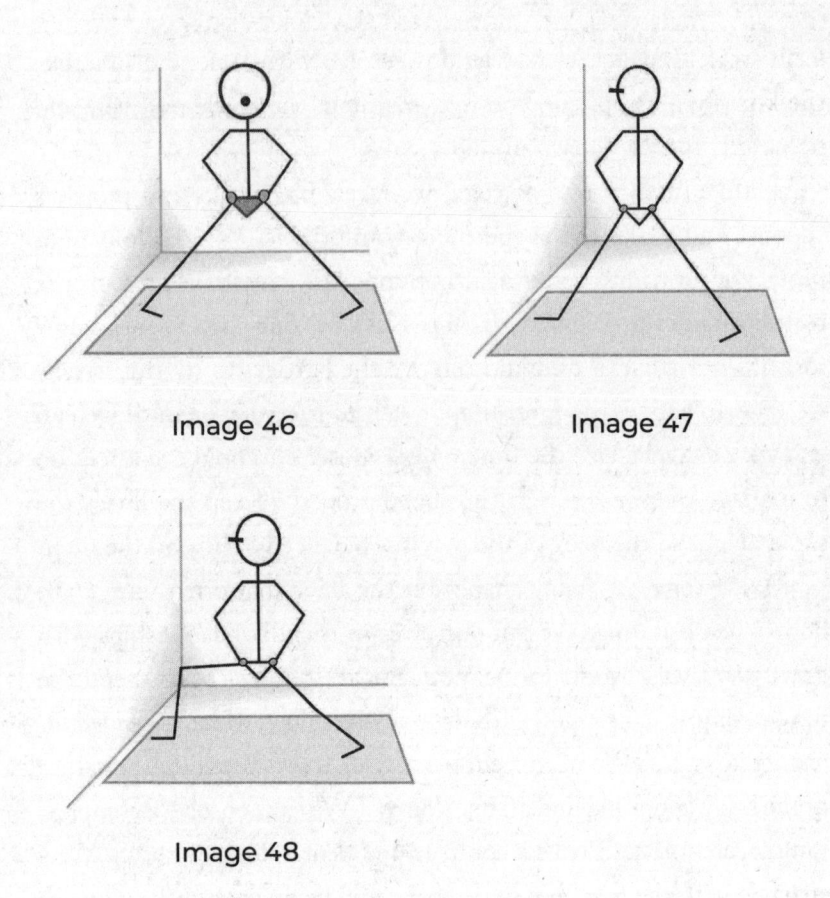

Image 47

Image 48

VIRABHADRASANA II

Warrior II

Hip Health

We use standing shapes for specific characteristics and qualities, but primarily to integrate our work on the floor. Getting predictable and lasting results in standing poses alone is almost impossible because the compensation patterns and restrictions we are trying to resolve are often used to support us in gravity. It makes it hard to identify and release them if they are being subconsciously relied upon.

Look carefully at the illustrations. The shape in Image 46 is a helpful counter position to the external rotation in Supta Baddha Konasana. In images 47 and 48, can you see the externally rotated hip in the front leg? Can you see the internal hip rotation in the back leg? Can you picture the compressive forces going through the knee and into the hip as the front leg bends? Can you see the depth of the work and the helpful practicality of a shape like this? There's so much going on in the lower body, we don't bother doing the fancy work with the arms and hands in the upper body. Including the arms shifts us away from the helpful depth in the legs and hips. There's also a tendency to "get it right" and become more performance-based. Keep your hands on your hip bones and let the work go to the lower body. We have plenty of shapes for the arms.

Standing with your legs wide, align the heels with the back edge of the mat and turn them out so that the toes point in. The stance is broad but not so wide that you can't effectively straighten the knees. Turn the tailbone down toward the floor, automatically moving the pubic bone toward the ceiling. Play with this for about thirty seconds to organize the body and feel the tissues adapting to the shape (Image 46).

Now, turn the right foot out toward 90° or as far as your hip will allow but no more than 90°, which means your toes point toward the wall to your right (Image 47). Remain here for another thirty to sixty seconds, firming your thighs, straightening your knees, and allowing your pelvis to adapt to the shape. We *do not* have any particular movement of the pelvis here. Don't pull the left hip back, and don't try to organize your body in a single plane. None of that, please. Pulling in old patterns from prior yoga will not aid in your healing. The work in your hips and lower back is happening with the addition of a very subtle downward movement of the tailbone.

If there is any pinch or pain in the lower part of your back or sacrum, shorten the stance or relax the pelvis. It's easy to get excited and push for more in shapes like this, but a particular outer ideal is risky to the hip and the sacroiliac joints. "Hip openers," as the term often goes, are dangerous because they oversimplify the approach to hip mobility. Hips get stuck in infinite ways, so we need many shapes to find and resolve them and their compensation patterns. The classic hip opener can sometimes create a problem where none existed. This can manifest as a torn labrum and/or hypermobility in the SI joints. Remember, hip and lower back movements coincide. Be kind to your body parts. They work together.

Next, press back through a straight left knee into the left heel and slowly bend the right knee in the same direction the right toe is pointing (Image 48). Hip rigidity and knee problems are intimately related, so don't force the moment or the movement. Let it reveal the issues. We'll address them more carefully on the floor in different shapes. Keep your eyes open and your hands on your waist. Move slowly and listen with your mind. Can you feel the pressure changes in and around the hip? If not, can you imagine them? Pay attention to the compressive forces inside the knee and behind the kneecap. Stop the movement if it gets frightening or painful. Is there a point in the shape where you can maintain it for another thirty to sixty seconds and allow the physiology to go to work in the knee, the hip, and the ankle? It's here that we re-organize your nervous system, muscles, bones, and joints to promote balance and a better walk. There is a lot going on, and being a little shaky in the shape is okay. It's good to feel your feet making hundreds of minor adjustments.

Straighten the right knee, turn the right toes in so that both heels point out, firm the tailbone down (bringing the pubic bone toward your nose), straighten the knees, relax your hands on your hips, and then repeat all the same details on the second side, turning the left foot out and the right toes in a bit. Be open to different sensations on the second side—always wary of the temptation to make one side symmetrical with the other.

Image 49   Image 50

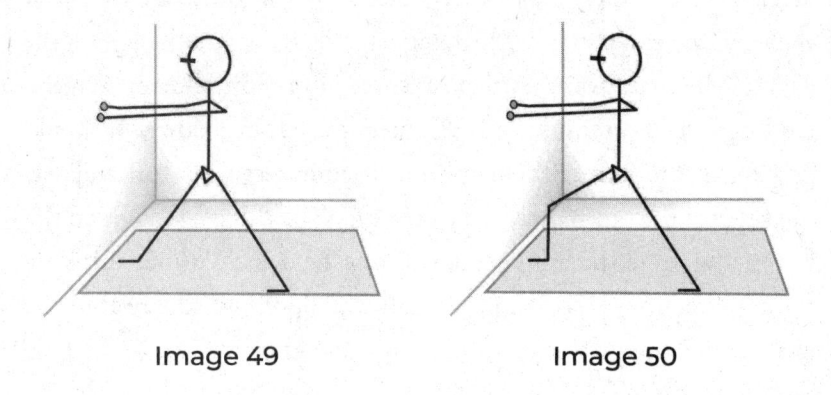

VIRABHADRASANA I
Warrior I
Foot, Knee, and Hip Movement

We need not be warriors to have a healthy walk. We don't need to take on the symbolism or attitude of the shapes or their names. Instead, let the healing yoga come to you as you experience each shape and the information it offers. Along with revealing compensatory patterns, the warrior shapes integrate our work on the floor by bringing the changes into practical upright movement. The hips, knees, and feet are designed for all kinds of movement that sitting, walking, hiking, and cycling cannot touch. We benefit from standing shapes to expose the greater potential of movement to keep hips, knees, and ankles vital and healthy.

To begin, place your right foot in the middle of the mat with your big toe close to the wall. Have your hands on the wall for support at shoulder height. Take a big step back with the left foot and line the left heel with the left edge of the mat. Pause and give your body a moment to adapt to the shape. If it feels unstable, shorten your stance. Now look down at your feet and turn each heel out an inch or two so that the outer edge of each foot is parallel to the edges of the mat. Pay particular attention to the left heel and shorten your stance if necessary so that the outer, lateral part of your heel is on the edge of the mat. You may feel resistance in the hip, knee, Achilles tendon, and/or calf muscles as you press the left heel down. It should be firm to the mat without too much effort. Pause again and feel the support of your hands and feet. Firm your thighs, straighten the knees, and press the left heel down into the mat. Without thinking about perfection, level the pelvis with the floor and square it to the wall. Look straight ahead, grow your spine long, and move the tailbone toward the floor (Image 49).

Hold for about a minute and slowly bend the right knee while keeping all the other details unchanged (Image 50). Keep the left knee straight and firm the left heel down. Sometimes we bring our hands to the waist, but not if it turns into a balancing act. Mobilizing the joints, reorganizing the nervous system, and integrating the muscles with this new mobility leads to better balance. Testing and wobbling do nothing for balance. When the work is over after another minute or so, straighten the front knee and release the shape. Repeat on the other side. Keep the shapes doable and sustainable.

Many variations of this shape bring health and mobility to the hips, knees, and spine. They are exaggerated but practical walking movements held in static "moments." They improve balance by putting a healthy demand on the feet and ankles to mobilize, strengthen, and integrate with the rest of the body. Can you see it in the illustration? Can you feel it in your body? These practical shapes integrate the floor work, expose restrictions, and improve your walk.

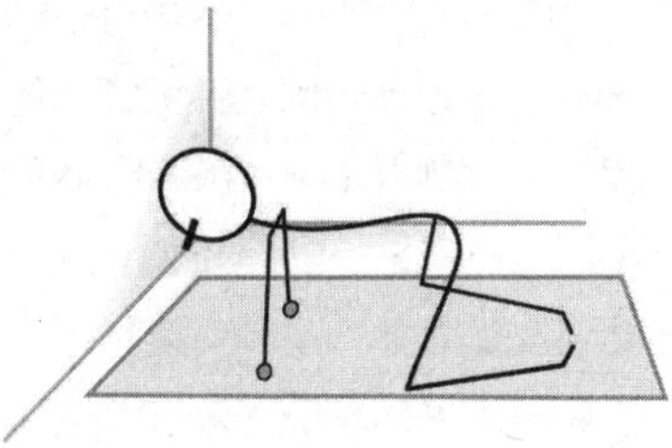

Image 51

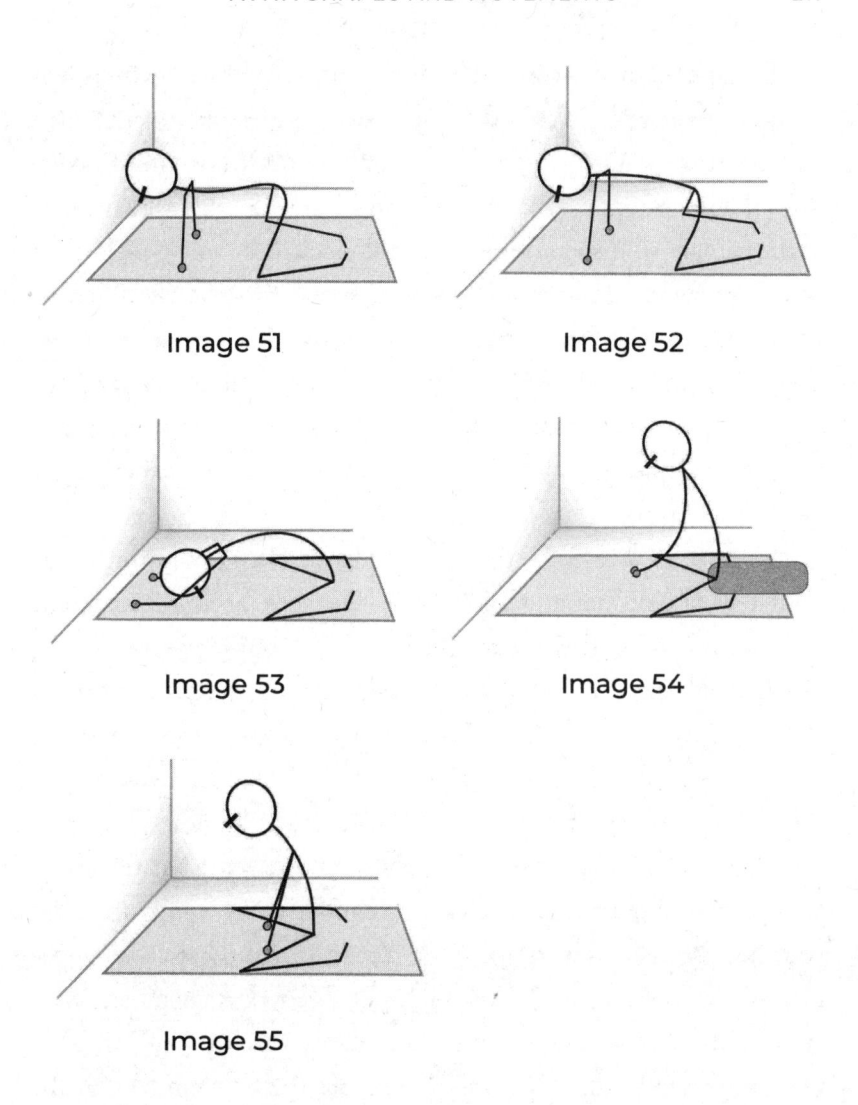

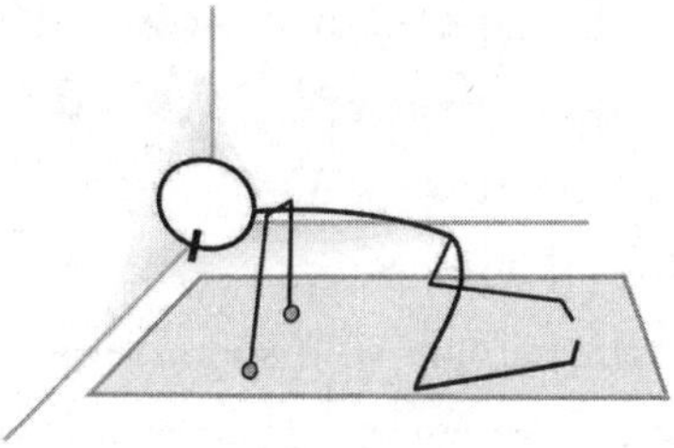

Image 52

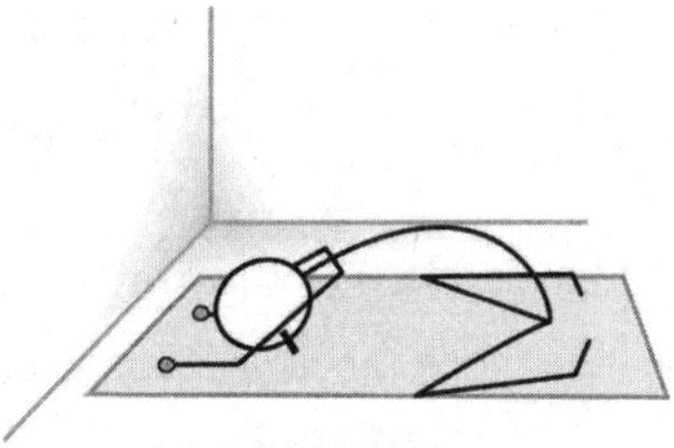

Image 53

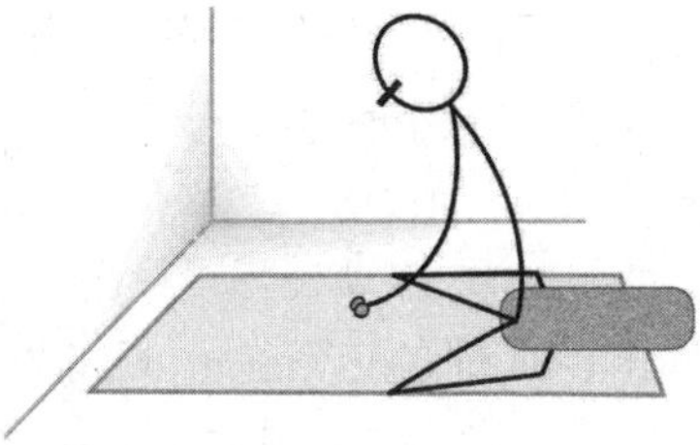

Image 54

Image 55

VIRASANA

Sitting On Heels

Flexion of the Knees, Feet, and Toes

Consider the image and experience of a cow resting in a pasture as you approach this shape. But remember, cows have been doing this shape for hours every day since birth. That cow, as long as it's able to kneel, will never have arthritis, knee pain, or hip problems.

Because humans search for comfort and alter the environment to meet our needs, we stop doing practical shapes like this. Consequently, if we want to regain movement and health, we must take a slow, pragmatic approach. Who can do shapes like this all day long? Tradespeople who spend time on the floor. Unless you're a plumber or carpet layer, you have no reason to spend time on the floor, so you'll need to start from scratch. Don't let the pain frighten you. Go slow and try to avoid evaluating your position. Follow the cues, but don't compare. It should look the way it does and not what you think it *should* look like. Can you manage the pressure so you experience a healing sensation?

Start on all fours with the knees and lower legs hip-width apart. Your toes should point straight back, and your heels should point toward the ceiling. Feel the weight equally on your hands and knees. Stop here (Image 51). What do you feel? Lift your belly and turn the tailbone down some (Image 52). That's the posterior rotation of the hip and flexion of the lumbar spine. It will change the sensation in the knees, the hips, and maybe even the feet and ankles.

Slowly sink back, moving the pelvis into the space between your heels. Keep your arms outstretched, shoulder-width apart, allowing your head to relax toward the floor. Your torso and belly also lower toward the floor between your thighs (Image 53). Remember, Avita cues are directional and not an end in themselves. They are intended to move you in a specific direction to expose the problems and instill healing compression.

Your work or *yoga* is to actively manage the depth of the shape so the sensation in the knees is sustainable. Move slowly, using your hands and arms for support, and don't get ahead of yourself. Fear is a restriction. Be patient and work with fearful thoughts like physical constraints by kindly observing them. As mentioned above, a combination of flexion and extension can be remarkably healing for many knee issues, including arthritis and degeneration. Steady compression restores and heals joints, whether through flexion or extension. One begets the other.

If this shape is doable and sustainable, consider walking your hands back and moving your torso into a more upright, relaxed position (Image 55). This will add considerable weight and compression to the knees, feet, and ankles, which means more feedback. Listen! Move slowly to welcome and work with the first sign of restriction you feel. The shape will advance *as* the restrictions are resolved with practice and faith.

Virasana has many variations. Sometimes the knees are wide, with the toes pointing in and the heels out. Other times we place the bolster under the pelvis for support (Image 54). However, I strongly encourage students to manage the sensation and shape by using their hands and arms for support—it's good for them too. It's risky to reach for support and rely on it when you're far better off using your hands and arms supportively. If your arms tire, reduce pressure, come out, and wait for the next shape. We sometimes work *with* the fatigue that shows up, but it must be doable and not painful. It must feel safe on all levels. Sometimes we keep the knees, feet, and ankles pressing together as we lower back to encourage mobility between the tibia and fibula, knee, and ankle. It all works together, and it works best when it moves the way it's supposed to. Can you see how Virasana resembles the long-lost squat? Can you see how this movement would help you get it back?

Image 56

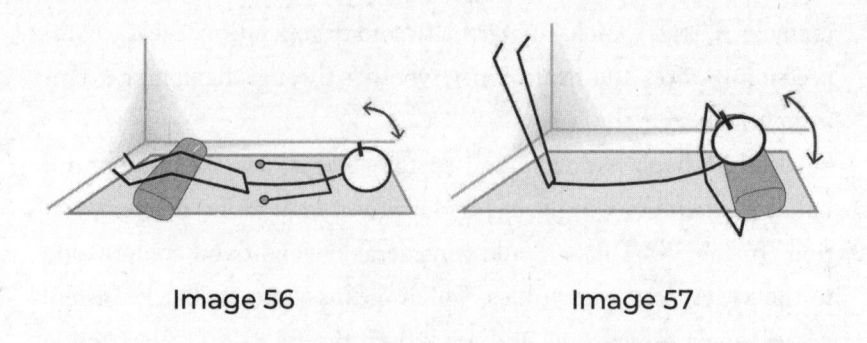

Image 57

SAVASANA
Relaxation, Integration, and Lower Back Release

A restful body is a reflection of a restful mind. Do we not practice to experience a peaceful presence? In Avita, we aim to go deep into rest and restoration. Deep yoga, deep rest. We want to reach the bones, joints, tissues, cells, and perhaps even the DNA, so the yoga continues to work for us long after we finish a class.

The shapes illustrated here have many variations, but the key is for the lower back and sacrum to be relaxed on the floor. At this point, the gentle head turns stimulate a more profound sense of calmness and relaxation. We don't look for restrictions in shapes like this as much as we look for and welcome inner stillness and calm. Following practice, we often experience love and light flooding the mind in a shape like this. There's nothing better. It's the healing goal we seek and we grow it within by giving it away throughout the day.

CHAPTER 16
Results of Practice

Avita is a results-driven practice. Why bother if you don't get results? Here is a short list of what I sometimes consider "by-products" of consistent practice.

IMPROVED MOBILITY

Increased mobility is something nearly anybody can attain from Avita. Instead of stretching muscles, we get to the core of the limitation, which is most often found in the bones, joints, and nervous system. We think of restrictions, blockages, and adhesions as physical conflicts that consistent practice can resolve, which results in increased mobility.

BETTER CIRCULATION

One of the causes of pain is reduced circulation.[63] As mobility improves, circulation improves, resulting in diminished pain. With better circulation, everything gets healthier, including muscle suppleness and tonicity. But Avita does more than improve the flow of blood. It encourages lymph flow throughout the body, strengthening the immune system.

A BETTER WALK

Increased mobility and range of motion give us more ways to live freely in our bodies. We walk better, dance better, and enjoy activities and sports with restored agility. If it's not your game that improves, maybe it's playtime with your kids or grandkids? Avita puts "the spring" back in your step; the practitioners I know seem to enjoy life a lot.

A BETTER SEAT

As we age, we tend to lose the mobility that allows us to sit in different ways. In turn, variations on the way we sit help inspire mobility. As we succumb to restrictions, the options for getting comfortable diminish, so by increasing mobility, we regain and maintain alternative ways to sit. You might regain the ability to sit on the floor or get up and down from a seated position with efficiency and ease. With improved balance and better hip and knee movement, you can get in and out of the car more easily or confidently sit on a bike seat and ride again.

BETTER BALANCE

Better mobility and balance reduce the risk of falling. One in ten people struggle with limited mobility, but that increases to four out of ten after age 65.[64] Trying to improve balance when mobility is absent does little good. Good balance comes automatically with increased mobility, leading to safer walking and a more agile way of life.

A BETTER REACH

We don't realize the importance of reaching overhead until we lose the movement. Reaching up and pulling a sweater over your head is practical, but extending the arms overhead is vital to shoulder health. A better reach means less shoulder pain and more circulation to the neck and head. Reaching high on your tiptoes to get that item off the top shelf is a sign of health and agility, and if you've lost it, you can get it back with Avita Yoga. We address mobility issues from fingers and shoulders to toes and feet, all necessary for the big overhead reach.

BETTER SLEEP

One of the most common by-products of the practice is that people sleep better. Why? Because they are more comfortable. There's less tossing and turning, and they have more time in one restful position. As the body reorganizes into a healthier balance and increased range of motion, it becomes easier to rest and sleep in multiple positions. We don't need to overexert and deliberately exhaust ourselves to sleep well. Improved mobility means less stress throughout the day, making for a more peaceful night. As the day goes, so goes the night. The brain gets better nourishment, circulation improves, and more oxygen helps maintain deep sleep.

A PEACEFUL PRESENCE

Until we confront "our stuff," we avoid the pain and the inner work of identifying and resolving the obstacles to health and happiness. We prefer to maintain familiar behaviors and attitudes, while managing our surroundings to help us feel good about ourselves. It's "easier" to continue on the well-traveled path, pursuing the people, places, and things we *think* bring happiness. We need a way not to pacify the mind but to heal it.

Our yoga is to slip below the surface and find the source. The Avita shapes and the purpose we give them will save you time, and your body will be the benefactor of its healing by-products along the way. A mobile body is helpful, but with a flexible mind, the possibilities are endless.

As we identify and resolve problems in the body, we unwind the past and slip into the healing power of Now. It's a productive and often enjoyable way to use a few hours of your week. If Avita is part of your life journey, I hope this book provides motivation and inspiration to practice.

CHAPTER 17

Quiet Breath, Quiet Mind

Perhaps you have heard about pranayama and breathing techniques to improve your health and facilitate your spiritual practice. Endless variations of the pranayama practice have developed over the years. Still, if we refer to the Yoga Sutras for insights on breathing, we find a simple suggestion in the first book. After several previous sutras that suggest ways of maintaining a calm mind, we get this one.

Sutra 1.34 Or that calm is retained by the controlled exhalation or retention of the breath.[65]

Here, Patanjali offers one of the few ancient insights on using breath to maintain a calm mind. We know that if the mind is calm, the body will follow. He suggests that a quiet state of mind is promoted and maintained by controlled exhalation or retention of the breath. He's making it simple for us.

Many breathing practices excite the nervous system to stimulate energy and create a feeling of bliss, which competes with a sweet, sustainable, undisturbed calm. The "buzz" is a side effect of hyperventilation, where carbon dioxide is expelled at an unhealthy rate. Overbreathing will not increase long-term oxygen levels or health. A CO_2 buzz is not enlightenment.

Exciting the system does not generate more energy, nor is it sustainable. We can become addicted to the buzz and the temporary high that come with aggressive yoga and pranayama. You may feel good afterward, but yoga is not a drug; yoga is a practice that helps us source peace and happiness so we can live gracefully, always. Drugs offer short-term "benefits" but may have long-term consequences. If your yoga practice is not sustainable in the short run, it will not be sustainable in the long run. Think deeply and honestly and ask yourself if your exercise program is working and sustainable. Is it something you will do in thirty, forty, or even fifty years to maintain health? If you are not sure, read on. Breath is a perfect barometer to help you enjoy all your favorite activities safely and sustainably.

Isn't it interesting that the yogis of long ago learned that the body and mind are calmed by controlling the exhale or retaining the breath? Today, we are led to think the opposite. Here is how conventional thinking goes: My body needs oxygen. If some oxygen is good, more is better. I get oxygen by breathing, so the more I breathe, the more oxygen I'll get.

But that's not how physiology works. Increasing the respiratory rate happens when we need to "take flight," as in running for our lives. This is the natural response of the sympathetic nervous system, and anything stressful or exciting will kick it in. It's lifesaving in the short term but has negative and potentially long-lasting consequences when overused. Increasing the breath while sitting still may be even worse. It stimulates the fight-or-flight mechanisms in the body, which excite the systems and dump a combination of stress-response hormones into the blood—but there's no reason to run and nowhere to go. To justify it, we spiritualize the breath and turn it into something magical and special, making the body real and drawing us away from the still, calm, healing power of Now found in the heart of the mind.

Excitability is not healing. It's the exact opposite of the rest and repose qualities of the parasympathetic nervous system.

We've been taught that CO_2 is a waste gas, but we need a certain level of CO_2 in the blood for healthy metabolic function. Did you know that increasing the body's tolerance for higher CO_2 levels enhances the unloading of oxygen into tissues to meet the oxygen demand at a cellular level.[66]

Though breathing less goes against conventional wisdom, you will experience the benefits with practice. Start slowly and see if you can learn to breathe only through the nose. If you must breathe through your mouth, find out why. Sometimes, the shift to nasal breathing will clear the resistance and stuffiness. It's the good ol' "use it or lose it" principle at work again. If you cannot breathe easily through your nose, one or both sides of the nose may have physical blockages. Consider consulting an Ear, Nose, and Throat specialist (ENT). There are simple procedures to improve nasal patency.

If you are athletic and enjoy pushing yourself, you may have to slow down or "start over" with a beginner's mind, which is not easy if you have a competitive drive. Contemplate the difference between fitness and health and get clear on which one you value most. The shift to nasal breathing can be challenging if you have been conditioned to operate under higher stress levels. With gentle willingness, you can learn to let the air flow only in *and* out of the nose in all activities and use it to regulate the intensity of your activity. Are you willing to slow down for better health? Decreasing intensity lowers the risk of injury and increases a mindful approach.

Like a simple walk in the park, Avita is a beautiful way to slow your pace and practice breathing less. With practice, your activity levels can increase while you maintain nasal breathing. I recommend *The Breathing Cure* by Patrick McKeown for more information on this topic. Patrick is an expert on the work of Dr. Konstantin Buteyko, a Russian pulmonologist tasked with discovering a way for cosmonauts to use less oxygen in space. Buteyko noticed that sick patients breathed rapidly and through their mouths, which prompted him to test his theories with his patients. Techniques to reduce breathing and isolate the breath through the nose were refined after experiencing positive results. Dr. Buteyko had two primary indicators for optimal health: a low pulse rate and a low respiratory rate. In practical terms, calm breathing is necessary to nurture and support healing.[67]

In the case of more breathing, we unwittingly work against the body's natural intelligence and push the physiology into imbalance. We cannot heal when sympathetic stressors are activated. Most people live out their day in stressful situations and then pursue activities like running or cycling as a cardiovascular workout to reach a point of exhaustion that results in a calm and relaxed feeling. Is it a substitute for a more profound and sustainable practice to reach a lasting sense of health and peace? Only the practitioner would know. There are many coping mechanisms for a compromised lifestyle.

We don't want to get unconsciously trapped in the day-to-day struggle for accomplishment. The Greeks understood this so well that they gave us the myth of Sisyphus to learn it. Each morning he awoke determined to push the boulder to the top of the mountain only to have it roll back to the bottom by nightfall. It's the story about the never-ending drive to succeed in a world where nothing lasts.

I raise these questions and values to be contemplated. It does not mean you shouldn't exercise vigorously if you enjoy it. It's *how* we practice and *how* we approach the stressors that matter most. If you are looking for a fresh start, consider using only nasal breathing as a way to pace your activity. Need to breath out of your mouth? Stop, rest, and start again.

Here are the Avita breathing guidelines based on my research and personal experience.

1. **Breathe in and out only through the nose.** Again, if there are nasal obstructions, consider visiting an ENT. The nose is designed to purify, humidify, and fortify the air with a gas called nitric oxide that further assists with exchanging gasses in the body and decreases inflammation. The nose naturally regulates the inhale and exhale, which aids CO_2 retention. Many have lost the ability to nose-breath, but you can get it back. I recommend reading any of Patrick's books including *The Oxygen Advantage* for additional advice for chronic breathing concerns.
2. **Go for a short walk and breathe only through the nose.** I recommend doing this alone because conversing destroys the practice of nose breathing. Notice what happens when you climb a short flight of stairs or walk up an incline. Pace yourself, and the body will adapt. In short, with practice, you will condition yourself to tolerate higher CO_2 levels, resulting in increased cellular health, decreased lactic acid build up, and increased stamina. We are going for long-term, sustainable health and a joyous life. Quiet breath, quiet mind. The body will follow.
3. **Practice on your mat with Avita Yoga.** We teach at a pace that allows you to breathe only through the nose, and Avita teachers will remind you. Don't make your breath loud, large, or audible. If you know about Ujjayi breath, understand that it is a more recent addition made by Krishnamacharia in order to help keep his students in sync as they performed vinyasa poses for an audience. Remember, less is more. If it becomes stressful, slow down and breathe normally in and out of the nose. Relax your jaw and face and

keep the focus where it belongs—in the details of the shape and the feedback it generates.
4. **Bring nasal breathing into all that you do.** You can even learn to stop sighing and yawning. Both are triggered by a buildup of CO_2, which you want to retain to enhance the exchange of gasses in the tissues. Instead of sighing or yawning, swallow and resist the temptation. The body will reorganize with practice, and the need for mouth breathing and yawning will abate. I resisted this suggestion when my wife, Lori, told me about it, but something clicked, and I dedicated myself to it. After one month the urge to sigh and yawn disappeared. If you carefully consider it, a sigh may be a complaint in disguise and is not necessary. Watch your body to watch your mind.
5. **Pause between the exhale and the inhale.** The amount of time you can peacefully pause before your next inhale is a good measure of well-being. With practice, you can advance to longer milestones. Longer, stress-free retention times and developing a willingness for air hunger will improve biochemistry. This physiological detail is known as the Bohr Effect, named after Christian Bohr, who was credited with the discovery in 1904.[68] Perhaps you remember studying it in high school science. Please refer to any of Patrick McKeown's books for more advanced techniques and a deeper understanding of physiology. How did I come upon all these insights about breathing? My wife, Lori, completed his training certification to help her dental patients with breathing issues.

This ancient yet scientifically proven breath awareness facilitates asana movement and centers the body and mind to source inner calm. This is just one more example of what makes Avita Yoga all-encompassing with physical and spiritual components that help you heal.

CHAPTER 18
Food for Thought

If you are using some time to give your bones and joints the pressure they love, why not nourish them and generate the best inner environment for success? If enjoyable, why not eat to reduce inflammation and supplement the healing physiology? It sounds good, but let's not get ahead of ourselves. While there are cause-and-effect relationships with the foods we ingest, the *beliefs* behind our food choices must be examined as well.

We've all heard the story about someone's grandma who lived to be one hundred years old on a diet that may not be deemed healthy. What we consume could be less important than our beliefs *about* what we consume. It is the power of belief that gives rise to the placebo effect. The mind is powerful beyond measure, so as I share some ideas about food to fortify your practice, do the inner yoga and watch the thoughts and feelings that come up as you read and experiment—they are important and must be resolved to free ourselves from food rules. Let's not give our healing power over to consumables but use our food choices as another helpful tool to maintain health and peace.

There's one universally helpful idea when it comes to food: Eat for the joy of it. But that's easier said than done. Can you eat and drink with no guilt and no shame? There's the yoga. Can you imagine how liberating it would be to unpack the memories, thoughts, and beliefs around beverages and *food*? Looking deeply at those can reveal a hidden attraction to the underling beliefs in lack, guilt, and fear. Doing the inner work to unwind the conditioning regarding consumption can be a massive part of the healing process.

Nutrition has been a favorite topic of mine for years, and I have experimented with my diet a lot. My high school senior thesis was a heartfelt paper on the ill effects of sugar on the body. I have food preferences, and I'm about to share them. There was a time when I made them food *rules*, and that didn't work because it got in the way of deeper meaning—like the time I provoked my girlfriend for ordering a Rum and Coke on our first date. But forgiveness saved the relationship, and she became my wife. Still, she won't let me forget it, and we enjoy a good laugh whenever we recount that delicate moment.

How can we make nutritional guidelines truly helpful? The same way as anything else: We use them to show us a better way by letting go of something that holds us back.

MEET GEORGE JETSON

Except for the flying cars, *The Jetsons* age is here. Do you know the cartoon? It was about a family living in the future and aired in 1962. My friend Steve and I treasured Saturday mornings because all three channels aired cartoons from 6 to 9 a.m. I'm sure I caught every episode as a young kid, but the only one I specifically remember is the episode where Jane (George's wife) went to the doctor with severe finger pain. She was diagnosed with *buttonitis*, and it was recommended that she take a break from all the "exhausting" button-pushing around the house.[69] We couldn't imagine such a condition in the 1960s, '70s, and '80s. It was funny. But today, almost everyone has buttonitis. I have done the yoga for my fingers, wrists, and shoulders almost daily to keep these parts happy and healthy over the five years at the keyboard creating this book.

Button pushing, typing, poking, mousing, swiping, and thumbing have brought a litany of upper body joint pains, including carpal tunnel syndrome and tennis elbow. Additionally, a lifestyle of button-pushing has contributed to nutritional complacency. We've traded deliberate food preparation and quality for efficiency and corporate profit. Many have lost the joy of cooking. We push buttons for food or have it handed to us by a food maker who also may have lost the love and joy of cooking. It's the way of the Jetsons, and the future is here.

Lifestyle efficiencies result from technological advances, but like anything in form, they come with costs. We get complacent and lazy, forgetting what real food looks and tastes like. The faster the food, the higher the refinement, which means less love and fewer nutrients. The farther we get away from the raw ingredients, the lower the quality of the ingredients. The result is a convenient product devoid of life and wholesome nutrients. Imagine someone saying, "I hate the taste of water," yet that is a statement my wife, Lori, heard often in her dental practice when she recommended drinking something other than soda. Have we become addicted to the taste of less healthy consumables? We have no idea what big business must do to mass-produce food, and it's been so ingrained in our lives that many don't care. We eat because it tastes good, not because we consider the nutrients our bodies want and need.

Avita Yoga goes well beyond symptom relief to resolve buttonitis. Still, it will work even better if you begin to question what you consume, get back to the roots, and do the work of nourishing yourself. Getting closer to the raw ingredients takes more time and effort than pushing buttons, but it's worth it. It's okay to slow down. In a world where food quality is diminishing, experimenting with diet is increasingly important. Question everything.

Most diet books are examples of what's worked well for the author and a cross-section of people who share a similar constitution, but no one diet works for all. We must experiment. Some people can eat a lot of anything and never gain weight. Others scrimp and count calories and can't seem to shed the pounds. That's why it's important to get to the thoughts and beliefs behind our attitudes about food.

What does the body do with all the junk we pour into it? It stores it. What it can't metabolize or eliminate gets tucked away. And what better place than fat? What if your body was generating fat as a storage bin for toxins? Could this be why people who cut calories alone still have trouble losing "weight"? I don't know. It's a theory, and I know I'm not alone in this thinking.

I am offering some guidelines that might help you experiment and take charge of what goes into your body. It's the same yogic self-care of watching our thoughts and beliefs. Why not watch what goes from hand to mouth? Whether food, thought, or action, is it helpful or harmful?

ENJOY REAL FOOD AND CLEAN WATER

What is real food? To find it, you have to get closer to the source. Sound familiar? The craving for quick, efficient satisfaction has evolved into a massive food industry that refines raw ingredients into ready-to-eat products. Grocery shelves are lined, aisle after aisle, with packaged goods that have had the nutritional life refined out of them. As we succumb to simplistic food choices, we lose the desire and ability to start from scratch with healthy raw materials to produce a nutritious meal. Even raw ingredients are being adulterated with chemicals and pesticides, which means it takes extra work to find suitable materials to cook with. But you can do it. Gardening and small farms are returning because people want to get closer to the land and grow what they eat. We are demanding organic in the grocery store, too, and this is changing how crops are grown.

It's estimated that 75 percent of Americans are chronically dehydrated because, on average, we drink 2.5 cups of water daily, which is not enough.[70] Any liquid other than water has some degree of diuretic characteristic that causes your body to eliminate fluids. Not only do we not drink enough water, but the water substitutes we consume are dehydrating. Try having a glass or two of water *before* you go for the coffee or tea. See how you feel after you hydrate. Your body was designed to utilize water. Period. It's needed for hydration as well as for ongoing cleansing. Clean water has become so rare that most need a good water purifier no matter where they live. It's worth it. Drink clean water often.

AVOID CHEMICALS

Most Americans today are burdened with a list of health problems ranging from heart disease and obesity to cancer and diabetes—and they could all be food-related problems. Yes, we know stress, activity levels, and genetics play a role, but let's focus on food now. It's not necessarily how much we eat. It's *what* we eat. Calorie counting works for very few, yet it's the method many lean on when managing weight. It's not a weight problem. Like the diseases mentioned above, the added weight is a side effect of the poisons and chemicals that find their way into our bodies. It's like flushing a wet wipe down the toilet. You're not supposed to do that because, unlike toilet paper, they don't "break down."

Chemicals do the same thing in the body because the body does not know what to do with them. They appear on the label as stabilizers, preservatives, natural flavorings, artificial sweeteners, flavor enhancers, food colorings, pesticides, fertilizers, polychlorinated biphenyls (PCBs), and persistent organic pollutants (POPs). They come into the body, do their damage, and then the body says, "What do I do with this? I can handle a little bit, but whoa. This is too much." The body's clean-up organs, including the liver and kidneys, can only take so much abuse before they falter. The system gets clogged. Eventually, the body tucks these toxic newcomers away where it's "safe" because it has no history with them. What better place to store them than in a fat cell? Of course, some toxins find their way into all kinds of tissues, but fat is a likely favorite. By the way, fat cells can get bigger or smaller, but they don't go away naturally.

A note of caution: Some consider toxic accumulation and storage in adipose tissue a safer alternative to "storage" in the blood. Toxic chemicals released into circulation during weight loss and cleanses can pose a severe health threat. Before changing your diet or exercise routine, seek medical advice or coaching, especially if you have a chronic disease or medical diagnosis.

LIMIT SUGAR CONSUMPTION

Sugar comes in many forms, some worse than others. Corn syrup is a cheap favorite found in many processed foods. Look for it and avoid it. Nearly 10 percent of the world population has diabetes because various forms of sugar find their way into processed foods.[71] As mentioned earlier, I wrote my high school term paper on the ill effects of sugar, and one of my favorite sources was a book called *Sugar Blues* by William Duffy. Written in 1975, it is still relevant and loaded with helpful information. One of the things that stuck with me was the disastrous effects of sugar in the joints, which can promote arthritis. Why not eat to support your Avita practice and its healing qualities?

Did you know that sugar consumption can produce psychological effects similar to cocaine? The "sugar high" can be addictive because it alters the mood, which leads to an unconscious desire for more sugar. One red Twizzlers will lead to another. A diet high in sugar can lead to obesity, insulin resistance, increased gut permeability, and inflammation. Manufacturers probably understand and appreciate our addictions and feed us accordingly by adding refined sugar and addictive consumables to products because we like them, purchase them, and thereby "ask" for them. It's why one in three Americans are prediabetic, and 80 percent of them are unaware of it.[72] You can find out if you are in this category by taking the simple hemoglobin A1C blood test, which measures your average blood sugar levels over the past three months. It could provide helpful feedback.

BEWARE "LOW SUGAR" OR "ZERO CALORIES"

Ironically, this suggestion follows the previous suggestion to limit sugar consumption. "Low sugar" usually means high chemicals. Of course, food can be healthy and low in sugar, but that's rarely the case when the manufacturer is compelled to label something with low sugar. Many low-calorie sugar substitutes like aspartame and saccharin are chemical compounds relatively new to the human body. What should it do with something it's never seen before? If it can't metabolize or eliminate it, where does it go? But the problem doesn't stop there. Sugar-free, no-calorie foods and beverages rarely contain any real nutritional value, and they are highly refined, which can often rank them high on the glycemic index even when they are low in added sugar. Don't be fooled by catchy slogans.

WATCH OUT FOR PLANT-BASED FATS AND OILS

Olive, avocado, and coconut oils have stood the test of time. However, many grain and seed oils (think safflower, rapeseed, corn, soybean), which are found in a wide variety of processed foods, are questionable. Most consider nut oils to be good and nutritious. Please do the research and decide for yourself.

Evidence suggests that plant-based oils, including all forms of margarine and other partially hydrogenated oils (PHOs), raise cholesterol levels.[73] But why? The impacts of PHOs on tissues and cells are less known, but studies show that these modified oils irritate skin and promote blemishes like acne.[74] If they do this on the outside, what are they doing on the inside? Healthy fats and oils are essential to maintaining healthy cell membranes. But what if we feed our cells poor substitutes like PHOs?

Here's my theory: PHOs irritate the lining of blood vessels and cause inflammation. What essential compound does the body call upon to repair inflamed blood vessels? Cholesterol. The body produces cholesterol to fix the damage from the oils we consume to lower cholesterol. I have known people with low animal-product diets, and they still have high cholesterol readings. Instead of reaching for a pill, let's get to the source.

Assuming that cholesterol is the problem is like making a fire truck the cause of the fire. Just because fire trucks keep showing up at fire scenes does not make them to blame. If your cholesterol is high, consider the possibility that something is irritating the lining of your blood vessels, causing your body to produce cholesterol and layer it along delicate blood vessel walls to repair the problem. Many have high cholesterol levels and follow a low-cholesterol diet. Others have "high cholesterol" but no plaque build-up in the veins and arteries. Could it be that cholesterol is not the problem?

GO BEYOND THE LABEL

Lobbyists constantly try to reduce the information we see on the foods we buy. Manufacturers know people are starting to read labels, so they find clever ways to hide information. You have to be a detective to find good food, or shop at one of the rare stores that do the work for you and commit to healthy ingredients, such as Natural Grocers. Back in the '90s, health food stores were just that, *health food* stores. But many have become "healthy looking" food stores. They present or package the food with unique labeling to make it appear healthy. Customers snatch it up, and profit margins increase. It takes more time, money, and effort to source healthy, non-GMO, organic food. Can you make it a priority, nevertheless? You are worth it.

MINIMIZE PROCESSED FOODS

Calorie counting is old school. We've known for years that many lean people eat two or three times that of heavier people. Could we be getting fat and unhealthy because we no longer consume real food? Want proof? Watch a movie or documentary from the 1950s, '60s, or early '70s, and look at how healthy and fit the people were. *Woodstock: Three Days That Defined a Generation* is the one we were watching when Lori pointed this out to me.

Not so long ago, people didn't count calories, and obesity was an anomaly. We had real food and clean water to drink. We didn't have to think about finding natural or organic food because chemicals hadn't polluted the soil. Most food was organic, and it was all GMO-free by default. Farms were small, and the Industrial Revolution and corporate business had yet to make their way into agriculture. Today, grocery store aisles are packed with manufactured, chemically loaded, nutritionally depleted food, mainly because food has become a money machine. It's more than vitamins and minerals the body needs. It's the enzymes and biological life that don't survive the refinement that are vitally important.

For optimal health, go beyond refined foods and consider eliminating refined beverages, including alcohol.

GO ORGANIC AND NON-GMO

If you think buying clean, organic food is costly and difficult, then purchasing the "cheaper" alternative food will be automatic. It's the impulse item that comes quickly without doing the work and informing yourself about what goes into your body. What's the cost of poor health? What's the cost of being malnourished *and* overweight? I know one thing for sure: Bones and joints don't like it. Watch your thoughts. I'm not being nice; I'm being honest because there is *always* a better way!

There are other costs to choosing cheaper, easier food. It's the cost of a lower quality of life, the side effects of which include diabetes, difficulty breathing, sleep apnea, bone and joint degeneration, inflammation, and the limited ability to move and enjoy life. There are no guarantees a chemical-free diet will avoid such calamities. Still, it's essential to understand the ramifications of the typical "no fuss" diet that has become our default. Taking this kind of responsibility can be fun! Lori and I enjoy sourcing good food and making meals from scratch. We have preferences, but there's no sweat if they're not met.

ENJOY THE FAT WITH THE PROTEIN

We've been taught to avoid fat. This propaganda came about when big businesses learned that they could make cheap, plant-based oils and package them as a substitute for butter. If you "can't believe it's not butter," there might be a good reason to look closer. As previously discussed, butter and animal fats are linked to cholesterol because they contain cholesterol! We need cholesterol, and the liver will produce what it needs if we don't get it in our diet. Of course, anything can be overdone, but nature has put the fat with the protein, and it has been eaten together for thousands of years. Whether from a nut, avocado, or a piece of bacon, fat was meant to be consumed with the protein it comes with. I'm not pitching any particular diet because no one diet will work for all. There are lots of reasons you may opt to be vegetarian or vegan. We're not here to change others but to heal ourselves.

NOURISH YOUR GUT

In nature, big things decompose to feed the small, which, in turn, nourish the big again. The dream of life is a massive recycling project humorously portrayed in *Hamlet*, Act 4, Scene 3, where Hamlet teaches Claudius that the worm is "the emperor of diet" because it always has the last bite. Nowadays, we know there are bacteria smaller than worms, and it's those bacteria that, in turn, become part of the nourishment in plants and animals, which makes its way back into the food chain. When we see the beauty of a natural forest full of plants and animals, we glimpse a snapshot of the not-so-beautiful recycling process in the background—consume or be consumed.

Watch Fantastic Fungi, *a 2019 documentary about a fun guy who dedicated his life to mushrooms and their importance in cleaning up and nourishing the world. Mushrooms are master recyclers and have medicinal properties.*

Our Earth contains numerous ecosystems (or biomes) on land and water, where the large is broken down into the small. On a macro level, they are essential for the planet's health; on a micro level, they are crucial for our good health. For inspiration, watch *Kiss the Soil* about your earthly biome and *Hack Your Health* about your inner biome. Both are important because they're interrelated. We have become bacterial-phobic and overzealous about disinfecting and "killing germs on contact." Are they so bad? Can you keep them all out?

Instead, consider befriending our tiny, mighty companions. We don't eat only for ourselves; we eat to feed the bacteria that live in the gut, providing the building blocks to nourish the body. You have heard about the "good and bad" bacteria in the gut, which has launched an industry based on prebiotics and probiotics designed to optimize gut health. You can do your research, but the big takeaway is that we eat to feed the microbiome within. Chemicals, sugars, and processed foods destroy the "good bacteria" because they create a toxic environment that feeds the "bad bacteria." Just like outer worldly ecosystems, when your inner ecosystem is upset, it leads to problems elsewhere.

What happens to pristine wetlands when chemicals are introduced? They die, but they can be brought back to health with proper care. Why not find out what foods the good bacteria like and feed them? The by-products or "waste" from the bacteria nourish us, and there is increasing scientific evidence that these by-products influence the chemistry that communicates with the brain.[75] The microbiome in the gut is alive, and it's telling you what it wants. This could be the origin of cravings. Some crave a healthy, low-sugar meal, while others crave more sugar. Have we become unwitting slaves to the microscopic "emperor" of the gut? Could our tiny, mighty companions be telling us what to eat? Search the internet for the worst foods for gut health, and you will find these repeat offenders: sugar, alcohol, processed foods, fried foods, gluten, and dairy.

In addition, watch for regular consumption of medications, especially antibiotics and non-steroidal anti-inflammatory drugs (NSAIDs) like aspirin, ibuprofen, and naproxen. They devastate the important microbiome and thus hurt the gut lining. While NSAIDs may reduce inflammation and pain, most studies indicate these drugs do little to promote healing.[76] "Bad bacteria" trigger disease, promote aging, and create an environment contributing to leaky gut syndrome (LGS), a condition worth learning about.[77] LGS occurs when bacteria and nutrients that are supposed to be absorbed through the villi and into the bloodstream instead pass through the gut lining and into the abdominal space, where they accumulate and get stored in fat. Less nutrients go to the body, and more toxic fat builds up inside the abdomen, limiting vital movement and motility of the organs within it.[78]

As discussed earlier, fat can accumulate to the point of restricting lumbar flexion and diaphragmatic movement, making it hard to breathe. Less movement means increased restriction and leads to a decrease in blood flow and health. Equipped with knowledge and peace as the goal, you can make healthier decisions without sacrifice! When the time is right, changes come quickly and easily.

What's your relationship with your gut? With more nerve endings than the spinal cord, it's often called the second brain. Perhaps a healthy intestinal bio system helps us make healthy and intuitive "gut" decisions.

SKIP A MEAL

Humans have not always had instant access to food and drinks. Convenience is a relatively new component of life here. What if the body, like that of many other animals, not only adapted to periods without food but thrived because of them?

For years, the thinking was to eat when you're hungry, and I subscribed to it; that approach works pretty well if you're eating real food and staying active. Still, recent trends about the benefits of fasting have been well established. Your body and digestive system need a break! My dad, taught me this when I was nine or ten. Modern studies show significant benefits when you stop eating for as little as sixteen hours. It's called intermittent fasting, and I recommend two books on the subject. Lori was inspired by *Fast Like a Girl* by Dr. Mindy Pelz, and I was drawn to *Fast This Way* by Dave Asprey, who gave us Bullet Proof Coffee—which I'm enjoying as this sentence comes through my fingers. While some may fast to lose weight, it seems that all may fast for the detoxifying effects for the body and mind. The more toxic your diet, the more careful you need to be. If you have a chronic disease or cancer, fasting may be beneficial, but you must get expert advice. Chronic problems and "diseases" may be far more related to the food we are eating than they are hereditary. I am no expert on food, and I do not give dietary advice. I can only share what works for me and the many I see.

As you experiment with nutrition and take up an Avita practice, you may go through unsettling periods as positive changes occur. Health and happiness are often preceded with some doubt and darkness. Sometimes it feels like time is speeding up and life gets more intense. It's normal and almost expected when any kind of deep undoing occurs. Hang in there. There is light on the other side. You may consider joining our chat forum to pose questions, share, and garner support. Again, I'm not suggesting you go against your doctor's orders, but it can be helpful to experiment.

Who is willing to take Socrates' advice to heart and examine your life to make it worth living?

CHAPTER 19
Know Your Constitution

Knowing your constitution and working within its limits is far better than trying to overcome it in an attempt to become someone you are not. The media is full of images and stereotypes suggesting that health has a particular look, and the medical model and conventional fitness paradigms back it up.

As you read the four sections below, see if you can pinpoint where you land on that spectrum. These categories are not new. However, the unique characteristics I describe have come to me through witnessing thousands of bodies and personalities in hundreds of shapes and classes.

These theories come from over forty years of personal yoga experience and working on many bodies as a trained Rolfer. But most of this knowledge comes from watching countless bodies move through over thirteen thousand hours of yoga instruction and asking students clarifying questions. Forever a student, I have wanted to know what others feel and why they feel it. It's how theories are transformed into sound practices. After a while, it all starts to come together, and we can learn to see the body and predict the blockages, the patterns, and the degree to which it will adapt to various yoga shapes. The Avita shapes are both informative and therapeutic.

THE FLEXIBLE CONSTITUTION— "I WANT TO FEEL MY BODY"

Those with a flexible constitution often seek sensation through increased intensity and a desire to advance the body. They gravitate toward gymnastics, dance, and contemporary yoga. They are revered for their physical prowess, which often tempts them to find new "edges." If this is you, watch for the tendency to make a flexible body *more* flexible. Like many, you may feel tightness in your muscles because they work harder to carry the load that should be in your joints and bones.

Those with a flexible constitution can become addicted to the stretch because it feels soooo good. Many will convey a need to *feel* their body, which can result in a continual push for more sensation. Unless they are injured or become disenchanted and stop the repetitious moves, the problems come later because elongated muscles can lead to disorganization and destabilization. With repeated attempts to perfect the pose or dance move, they unwittingly avoid the few restricted areas as the loose parts are overused and become looser. Sometimes the problem is brought to the surface later in life when hormonal shifts occur and the career comes to a close.

Can you see how more stretching could be harmful and sometimes painful to a flexible constitution? Would adding flexibility to an already flexible body be helpful? These people need stability, and along with finding and resolving the few restricted areas, Avita yoga can help. I also appreciate Pilates for flexible people. Joseph Pilates opened his first location next door to a dance studio to help generate stability for dancers. It was so effective and inspirational that some of the early dancers went on to teach Pilates to help prevent injury in the dance population.

Avita Yoga is most challenging to those with a flexible constitution because it requires muscular work to which they are not accustomed. However, it can reorganize the systems to transfer the effort from the muscles to the bones where it belongs. Even the passive shapes will require some effort to keep the focus on the reorganization and not on the easy "yin quality" that flexible people prefer. It will take a little time and determination because it also involves reorganizing the nervous system. But with practice, the transfer does come. They feel more integrated, and the seemingly vital need to push and *feel* their body disappears. Avita is great for this type of constitution, but it will feel like work as you create more stability and slowly take the demand off your muscles.

THE TIGHT CONSTITUTION— "I'M NOT FLEXIBLE ENOUGH"

On the other end of the spectrum, stiffer people are wired tighter, which moves the supporting mechanism into the structural components of the bones and joints. They don't necessarily feel stiff until they move into a shape or position that reveals the limitation, so they shy away from things like yoga, dance, and gymnastics.

Bodies on this tighter end of the spectrum provide ample feedback, so instead of seeking more sensation, they tend to avoid it altogether. Most yoga styles overwhelm their system. They tend to experience stiffness closer to the joints and "in the bones." If you are on the stiffer side, the thought of stretching is usually appalling—and for good reason.

Stretching the muscles is not only painful and unpleasant for these types of bodies, it misses the problem. These people benefit by targeting joint restrictions that lead to an undoing of patterns, both physically and neurologically. Passive shapes tend to come readily and without effort for rigid people, although they will need to actively support the shape at times. The muscles release automatically as these bodies tend to quickly drop into the bones and joints where, along with the nervous system, reorganization occurs. It feels good to them. With practice, they feel more mobile and pick up activities they once thought inaccessible.

As they drop into their bones and joints, they are often surprised at how good it feels. Some start to practice more frequently as the changes come. If this describes you, I invite you to let the unwinding begin. Avita is fantastic for this type of body.

THE ATHLETIC CONSTITUTION— "I CAN DO ANYTHING"

Athletic bodies are naturally organized. The nervous system is well balanced with the structure and the soft tissues. It takes unusual, significant, and sudden movements to cause injury. Agility and coordinated movement come readily and efficiently to the athletic body that tends to land in the middle of the spectrum. Combined with the fact that we all want to get better at what we're good at, it's no surprise that athletic constitutions excel in their activity or sport of choice. The competitive edge is almost always more mental than physical at high levels of expertise and professionalism, because athletic bodies can be finely tuned.

There are countless examples of this constitution, but think Lebron James and Caitlin Clark. Their bodies will do just about anything they ask. Can you see how they are weighted equally between flexibility and stiffness? We love watching them at their craft—so much so that we are willing to pay for it. The problem occurs when we idolize them as a perfect image and work toward being more like them regardless of *our* constitutional limits. It's risky business.

Understanding the difference between flexibility and mobility and where you fall on the spectrum is extremely helpful in managing expectations and the results you attain from various activities.

We may be amazed at the beauty of another's athletic ability, but we need not be awed by it. You may be inspired, but don't be envious. That is not a healing mindset. We each came in with unique hardware and software. Therefore, each must work with what they have, knowing that the more we specialize in our activities, the more we need the yoga. As accomplished as we may become in any given sport or activity, staying "out of the groove" is crucial to keep the bones and joints healthy. All too often, it's a strength and stretch approach alone that athletes rely on—and that's not enough.

PUTTING IT ALL TOGETHER— "I WANT PEACE OF MIND"

Can you begin to see that the inner experience of one's body, its constitution, and its ability to move is not only structural but also a product of the nervous system?

Flexible constitutions have more space in and around the joints, so the brain must innervate the muscles more to hold the body upright and keep it functioning.

In tight constitutions, the skeleton naturally supports the body, which means the nervous system may read various pains and trigger points, but the muscles don't always *feel* tight for these people. Because their bones and joints share a higher percentage of the load, they are not under constant demand to support the body as in a more flexible person.

Athletic constitutions, by comparison, have more ease of coordination between the muscles and the skeleton. Natural efficiency and balance allow these bodies to perform well with fewer problems unless they push to the point of injury.

I share this so you can befriend your body and take a wise, if not less traveled, path, and in hopes that you might ask better questions. I want you to know there is a reason for not wanting to stretch. If yoga, a particular self-care program, works for your friend but not for you, there's no need to force it. While I feel Avita is a revolutionary and, in many ways, timeless approach to yoga, I don't expect everybody to be drawn to it. Avita is *very* different.

Fascia also plays a massive role in bodily constitution. It holds us together and is loaded with nerve endings that inform the brain of our movements and spatial location. Can you see the importance of working with fascia? It supports us structurally, informs us proprioceptively, and is concentrated around the joints. Thus, our stiffness or tightness may not be so much of a hardware problem as *a software problem*. And we're born with it. We must be careful about looking for solutions where they don't exist. But if we understand and practice within our "constitutional boundaries," we can lead healthy, happy, and peaceful lives.

Above all, make no assumptions about flexibility and your yogic abilities. Take a kind and gentle entry. Come with a beginner's mind and leave your preconceived ideas about flexibility and yoga behind. Most have never considered their constitution and how it influences their approach to life and their decisions.

When you experience a stretchy sensation in a muscle, do it in a way that gives it time to communicate with the brain and the rest of the body. You may enter an Avita shape that feels "stretchy," but we never push to the point of stretching it. We wait. We trust. We use time and healing sensation in the position to allow communication between the tissues and systems. We use the feedback to interact with the subconscious mind and initiate a release to create practical agility.

CHAPTER 20
Know Your Inner Rhythm

We each have an inner rhythm accompanying us in our walk through life. Bodies "on the go" have a rhythm different from those who stop to smell the roses. No rhythm is better than another, but knowing your inner energetic rhythm can be helpful, especially when establishing a practice to rejuvenate your body and heal your mind.

There are countless ways to calm the mind, but even if you succeed at calming the tiger in your house, you *still* have a tiger in your house. Avita Yoga takes a different approach. We don't seek to calm the mind. We aim to heal it. Where are the shadows when we bring them to the light? There's a difference between placating a symptom and getting to its source, where it can be cured. As the obstacles to peace are washed away, the mind becomes and will eventually remain consistently calm. With practice, the day will come when, no longer attracted to the ego's temptations, you can relax and easily return to your center and the Source of lasting joy. We soon realize there's no other way to *be* and nothing is worth the cost of lost peace and happiness.

To the ego, it sounds boring, but anyone who has done the yoga can attest that life becomes a joyous adventure as we cleanse the darkness from our minds. And when the inner critic jumps in with its destructive analysis, we learn to give it up too. We observe *from* the healed mind, which lets its healing life force come *through*. We forgive and release everything that works against our healing—a journey-less journey to a reality we never left. Without judgment, the unhelpful patterns and problems disappear, and in doing our yoga, we unite with Source and experience a happy dream.

We bring our minds into the practice by watching the shape and the information that comes with it. For a fast-paced mind, this is not easy but it is essential. Some students are so anxious they can only endure the first fifteen minutes of class at first, and that's okay. Nothing forced will work. The Avita pace is slow, giving tissues time to respond and the mind time to soften. If you are fast-paced and athletically motivated, give it a chance. We all slow down eventually, so why not practice for a smooth landing?

A fast-paced mind is often associated with a fast-paced body, but the correlations can be all over the map. Like a cat purring in the sun, rhythm is the inner meditation that settles us deeply into the joined experience. Here are some questions that will help you find your healing rhythm. Quick answers are not necessary. Let the questions bring insights.

- Observe your rhythm or pace the next time you're out for a walk, either by yourself or in an activity with other people. How is your energetic rhythm different? Is it possible to hurry or "keep up" and simultaneously be peaceful?
- When walking, do you prefer to stroll or "burn calories"? Is there an agenda, or can you slow down and see the beauty in all things? What about your thoughts? Can you watch them "from a distance" without judgment?

- Are you competitive? Do you compete with yourself, or do you tend to look around for someone to catch and then pass up? Are you always out in front?
- Can you slow down and be okay? If not, why? Are you running *from* something? Are you running *toward* a mirage?

Often we avoid slowing down because it lets feelings of anxiety, lack, and fear come to the surface. But this is why we must start to slow down. Let those feelings rise so you can discover the truth: There is *nothing* to fear. Slow down, turn, and face the fear with love by your side. Something to gain means something is lacking, and *nothing* is lacking. Be here now and let peace be your goal and guide.

While there is movement, the Avita shapes require you to slow down. Could it be an inroad to a long-wanted meditation practice? If your pace is quick, try a shorter thirty-minute class, or just put your legs up the wall to help you stop and drop, if even for a moment. There's no proper meditation position. We use the shapes to throw the ego a bone to have a moment of peace and gentle release. We practice peaceful moments until peace is all there is.

NAMASTE

And now we say, "Namaste." It is a word often used as a salutation, and it's how I close the classes I teach. It's a beautiful word with positive connotations. But at its best, Namaste represents something eternal and beyond all error.

Namaste means seeing the love and light in others as a reflection of the same in ourselves. In this way, we learn to "see" with the heart, not the eyes. If there is only one Love, then the desire to join with it becomes the purpose of our relationships. Whether it's a heartfelt glance or smile to someone in the grocery line, navigating a challenging work relationship, or doing the profound inner work with a lifelong partner, namaste is practice. No relationship is too small or big, for seeing the sameness in all reduces social hierarchy and status to our common denominator. Seeing the Innocence beyond the words, actions, and body of another is required to see it in myself. It's healing. We join in the *only* thing we all have in common—love.

The Buddha discovered and taught a way out by acknowledging that the human condition is a life of suffering. How do we make that leap? We practice. We release the thoughts that uphold suffering and see through the lens of joined love in all we do. Like kids scuffling in a sandbox, we no longer have the sand in our faces when we "stand up" and stop buying into the drama. The sand may swirl around our ankles, but where's the conflict when seen from a higher state? In the healed mind, we are free.

In 2024, Lori and I joined a medical mission in Nepal. We enjoyed the opportunity to be with the people for a moment in time. The Nepali people use "namaste" as their greeting while looking you in the eyes. The greeting is a pause to say, "I see you, I love you, I am you."

All we need is provided, and everything we do and say is guided. We don't look back; we don't anticipate the future. Yoga is *now*, and now we practice.

Namaste.

ACKNOWLEDGMENTS

I want to thank those who have helped me along my path and made Avita and this book possible. To me, they are all teachers.

My first teacher was my dad. Thank you, James P. Bailey, DVM. He taught me how to care deeply and see through the eyes of others. He taught me the difference between thinking critically and critical thinking. Only the latter can lead to healing. He taught me the value of conservation and a conscientious approach to life. He taught me how to fix just about anything. We didn't throw anything away; we fixed it. Side by side, we had our hands in and on the bodies of his furry, four-legged patients, and here, I learned about muscle, innervation, and the body's ability to heal. Thank you, Dad.

Thank you to my mom, Beverly Bailey, OT, for her saintly generosity and kindness. She taught me how to have faith in God and gave me a keep-moving-forward attitude.

Thank you to my sisters, Mary Jo, RN, and Jennifer, CPA, for being patient with me.

Thank you, Dr. Norman Allard, my first yoga teacher, who planted the seed of the meaning of yoga and taught me the importance of never-ending research.

Thank you to the many talented, forward-thinking teachers at the Rolf Institute®, including Jan Sultan, Jim Asher, Gail Olgren, and Pedro Prado. You taught me about patterns and how they affect us. You taught me how to use my eyes and hands to see below the surface.

Thank you, Tom Meyers and Gil Hedley, for your inspirational anatomical insights. You helped me understand the vital role of fascia in our bodies and how to work with it to bring helpful long-term changes. You inspired me to have fun sharing anatomical insights with students and those who want to teach Avita.

Thank you, Reverend Gene Langlois, for setting the stage for a working marriage, marrying my wife and me, coauthoring my first book, *The Yoga Mind*, and being a teacher of love. I'm grateful to many other spiritual teachers, including Lynn Corona and Ken Wapnick, for their teachings and demonstration of clarity and purpose.

Deepest gratitude to my wife, Lori Kemmet, DDS, for supporting me in every endeavor. Many of the insights for Avita Yoga came through the world of dentistry and CE courses we attended together. Knowing that the script is written, we have learned there are no mistakes, and it's impossible to "mess it up." Your loving support makes life a fantastic and joyful adventure, and I'm grateful for it. You're a pretty good editor too.

Thank you to our child, Sunny "Georgia" Bailey, for being you. I appreciate your sincere empathy and passion for inclusivity for all people, including the LGBTQ community. You have been one of my greatest teachers.

Finally, I must thank my students and Avita teachers, who have inspired me to grow and share Avita Yoga so that others may heal. Thank you for your feedback, compassion, trust, laughing at my jokes, and willingness to go along with me on this giant experiment that, in many ways, contradicts everything we ever learned about the body and the mind. This willingness and trust are what make our relationships meaningful. We heal together or not at all.

NOTES

1. Dr. Ida Rolf Institute®, "The History of Rolfing®," https://www.rolf.org/history.php.
2. William Shakespeare, *Hamlet*, act 3, scene 1.
3. A Course in Miracles, "The Illusion and the Reality of Love," https://acim.org/acim/chapter-16/the-illusion-and-the-reality-of-love/en/s/205?wid=search&q=your%20task%20is%20to%20.
4. *Star Wars: The Empire Strikes Back*, directed by Irvin Kershner (1980; Los Angeles: Lucasfilm), film.
5. A Course in Miracles, "T-6.V-A.5:3," https://acim.org/acim/en/s/103#5:3.
6. W Brinjikji et al., "Systematic Literature Review of Imaging Features of Spinal Degeneration in Asymptomatic Populations," https://pmc.ncbi.nlm.nih.gov/articles/PMC4464797/.
7. D Purves et al., "Mechanoreceptors Specialized for Proprioception," https://www.ncbi.nlm.nih.gov/books/NBK10812/.
8. "In brief: What are ligaments?" https://www.ncbi.nlm.nih.gov/books/NBK525790/.
9. Cleveland Clinic, "Muscles of the Human Body," https://my.clevelandclinic.org/health/body/21887-muscle.
10. "In brief: What are tendons and tendon sheaths?" https://www.ncbi.nlm.nih.gov/books/NBK525770/.
11. National Institute of Arthritis and Musculoskeletal and Skin Diseases, "What Is Bone?" https://www.niams.nih.gov/health-topics/what-bone.

12. P Juneja et al., "Anatomy, Joints," https://www.ncbi.nlm.nih.gov/books/NBK507893/.
13. NASA, "Walk the Line: NASA Studies Physical Performance After Spaceflight," https://www.nasa.gov/humans-in-space/walk-the-line-nasa-studies-physical-performance-after-spaceflight/.
14. A Nahian et al., "Histology, Periosteum and Endosteum," https://www.ncbi.nlm.nih.gov/books/NBK557584/.
15. N Rosenberg et al., "Osteoblasts in Bone Physiology—Mini Review," https://pmc.ncbi.nlm.nih.gov/articles/PMC3678809/.
16. S Teitelbaum, "Osteoclasts: What Do They Do and How Do They Do It?" https://pmc.ncbi.nlm.nih.gov/articles/PMC1851862/.
17. Office of the Surgeon General, "3 Diseases of Bone," https://www.ncbi.nlm.nih.gov/books/NBK45506/
18. R Oftadeh et al., "Biomechanics and Mechanobiology of Trabecular Bone: A Review," https://pmc.ncbi.nlm.nih.gov/articles/PMC5101038/.
19. T Tamer, "Hyaluronan and synovial joint: function, distribution and healing," https://pmc.ncbi.nlm.nih.gov/articles/PMC3967437/.
20. A Seidman et al., "Synovial Fluid Analysis," https://www.ncbi.nlm.nih.gov/books/NBK537114/.
21. Physio-Pedia, "Synovium & Synovial Fluid," https://www.physio-pedia.com/Synovium_%26_Synovial_Fluid.
22. J Levick, "Microvascular architecture and exchange in synovial joints," https://pubmed.ncbi.nlm.nih.gov/8748946/.
23. M Null et al., "Anatomy, Lymphatic System," https://www.ncbi.nlm.nih.gov/books/NBK513247/
24. University of Michigan Health, "Difference Between Osteoarthritis and Rheumatoid Arthritis," https://www.uofmhealth.org/conditions-treatments/cmc/difference-between-osteoarthritis-and-rheumatoid-arthritis/.
25. National Institute of Arthritis and Musculoskeletal and Skin Diseases, "Osteoarthritis," https://www.niams.nih.gov/health-topics/osteoarthritis.

26. Advanced Bone & Joint, "Degenerative Joint Disease vs. Arthritis," https://www.advancedboneandjoint.com/2018/09/14/degenerative-joint-disease-vs-arthritis/.
27. Mayo Clinic, "Arthritis: Symptoms and Causes," https://www.mayoclinic.org/diseases-conditions/arthritis/symptoms-causes/syc-20350772.
28. Mayo Clinic, "Fibromyalgia: Symptoms and Causes," https://www.mayoclinic.org/diseases-conditions/fibromyalgia/symptoms-causes/syc-20354780.
29. C Galvez-Sánchez et al., "Psychological impact of fibromyalgia: current perspectives," https://pmc.ncbi.nlm.nih.gov/articles/PMC6386210/#:~:text=Vulnerability%20factors%20in%20fibromyalgia,and%20physical%20abuse%20and%20neglect).
30. Ibid.
31. Cleveland Clinic, "Degenerative Disk Disease," https://my.clevelandclinic.org/health/diseases/16912-degenerative-disk-disease.
32. Selina M. Parry and Zudin A. Puthucheary, "The Impact of Extended Bed Rest on the Musculoskeletal System in the Critical Care Environment," *National Library of Medicine*, PubMed Central, October 6, 2015.
33. Medical News Today, "Z-Scores for Bone Density," https://www.medicalnewstoday.com/articles/z-scores-for-bone-density-chart.
34. ScienceDirect, "Trabecular Bone Structure and Function," https://www.sciencedirect.com/topics/immunology-and-microbiology/trabecular-bone.
35. J Kim et al., "Osteoblast-Osteoclast Communication and Bone Homeostasis," https://pmc.ncbi.nlm.nih.gov/articles/PMC7564526/.
36. Y Lu et al., "Twelve-Minute Daily Yoga Regimen Reverses Osteoporotic Bone Loss," https://pmc.ncbi.nlm.nih.gov/articles/PMC4851231/.
37. L Fishman, "Yoga for Osteoporosis," https://journals.lww.com/topicsingeriatricrehabilitation/fulltext/2009/07000/yoga_for_osteoporosis__a_pilot_study.9.aspx.

38. B Bordoni et al., "Anatomy, Fascia," https://www.ncbi.nlm.nih.gov/books/NBK493232/.
39. C Crone, "Reciprocal inhibition in man," https://pubmed.ncbi.nlm.nih.gov/8299401/#:~:text=Reciprocal%20inhibition%20is%20the%20automatic,the%20control%20of%20voluntary%20movements.
40. National Strength and Conditioning Association, "Muscle Growth and Adaptation," https://www.nsca.com/education/articles/kinetic-select/muscle-growth/.
41. BYU Learning Center, "Function of Muscle Tissue," https://content.byui.edu/file/a236934c-3c60-4fe9-90aa-d343b3e3a640/1/module7/readings/function_muscle_tissue.html.
42. "Elasticity" definition, Britannica, https://www.britannica.com/science/elasticity-physics.
43. ScienceDirect, "Reciprocal Inhibition in Engineering," https://www.sciencedirect.com/topics/engineering/reciprocal-inhibition.
44. Ibid.
45. Medical News Today, "Rigid Muscles and Fibromyalgia," https://www.medicalnewstoday.com/articles/rigid-muscles#fibromyalgia.
46. Cedars-Sinai, "Swayback Lordosis Condition," https://www.cedars-sinai.org/health-library/diseases-and-conditions/s/swayback-lordosis.html.
47. Somatic Movement Center, "Pandiculation and Muscle Release," https://somaticmovementcenter.com/pandiculation-what-is-pandiculation/.
48. Philip Anloague, "Stiff Muscles as a Counterintuitive Superpower of NBA Athletes," The Conversation, May 16, 2019.
49. Nature Education, "The Sliding Filament Theory of Muscle Contraction," https://www.nature.com/scitable/topicpage/the-sliding-filament-theory-of-muscle-contraction-14567666/.
50. A Ferlinc et al., "The Importance and Role of Proprioception in the Elderly: a Short Review," https://pmc.ncbi.nlm.nih.gov/articles/PMC6853739/.
51. Psychology Today, "Neuroplasticity: The Brain's Capacity for Change," https://www.psychologytoday.com/us/basics/neuroplasticity.

52. G Wittenberg, "Experience, Cortical Remapping, and Recovery in Brain Disease," https://pmc.ncbi.nlm.nih.gov/articles/PMC2818208/.
53. Khan Academy, "Signal Propagation and Neural Synapses," https://www.khanacademy.org/test-prep/mcat/organ-systems/neural-synapses/a/signal-propagation-the-movement-of-signals-between-neurons.
54. B Bordoni et al., "Anatomy, Fascia," https://www.ncbi.nlm.nih.gov/books/NBK493232/.
55. P Kamrani et al., "Anatomy, Connective Tissue," https://www.ncbi.nlm.nih.gov/books/NBK538534/.
56. Ibid.
57. L Chang et al., "Anatomy, Cartilage," https://www.ncbi.nlm.nih.gov/books/NBK532964/.
58. Kyeong Min Son, Jeong Im Hong, Dong-Hyun Kim, Dae-Gyu Jang, Michel D. Crema, and Hyun Ah Kim, " Absence of Pain in Subjects with Advanced Radiographic Knee Osteoarthritis," PubMed Central, September 29, 2020, https://pmc.ncbi.nlm.nih.gov/articles/PMC7526196/.
59. Dr. Ida Rolf Institute®, "Structure and Function Journal," https://www.rolf.org/docs/structure_function_integration_journal_of_the_dr_ida_rolf_institute_digital_mar_2019_final.pdf.
60. Avance Care, "Polyvagal Theory and the Nervous System," https://www.avancecare.com/polyvagal-theory-your-nervous-systems-wiring-for-safety-and-connection/.
61 Rohit Jayakar, Alexa Merz, Benjamin Plotkin, Dean Wang, Leanne Seeger, and Sharon L. Hame, "Magnetic Resonance Arthrography and the Prevalence of Acetabular Labral Tears in Patients 50 Years of Age and Older," National Library of Medicine, August 2016, https://pubmed.ncbi.nlm.nih.gov/27098353/#:~:text=Materials%20and%20methods:%20From%202004,a%20more%20appropriate%20imaging%20tool.
62. Mayo Clinic, "Swollen Lymph Nodes: Symptoms and Causes," https://www.mayoclinic.org/diseases-conditions/swollen-lymph-nodes/symptoms-causes/syc-20353902.

63. Medical News Today, "Common Symptoms of Various Conditions," https://www.medicalnewstoday.com/articles/322371#symptoms.
64. Centers for Disease Control and Prevention, "Disability and Health Data System (DHDS)," http://dhds.cdc.gov.
65. P Tigunait, "Yoga Sutra 1.34," https://yogainternational.com/article/view/yoga-sutra-1-34-translation-and-commentary/.
66. A Benner et al., "Physiology, Bohr Effect," https://www.ncbi.nlm.nih.gov/books/NBK526028/#:~:text=The%20Bohr%20effect%20describes%20red,delivery/release%20at%20peripheral%20tissues.
67. Patrick McKeown, *The Oxygen Advantage: The Simple, Scientifically Proven Breathing Technique for a Healthier, Slimmer, Faster, and Fitter You* (William Morrow, 2015).
68. A Benner et al., "Physiology, Bohr Effect," https://www.ncbi.nlm.nih.gov/books/NBK526028/#:~:text=The%20Bohr%20effect%20describes%20red,delivery/release%20at%20peripheral%20tissues.
69. *The Jetsons*, season 1, episode 22, "Sad Jetsons: Depression, Buttonitis, and Nostalgia in the World of Tomorrow," aired March 3, 1963, Hanna-Barbera.
70. Taylor, Kory; Jones, Elizabeth B., "Adult Dehydration," National Library of Medicine, October 3, 2022, April 26, 2024. https://www.ncbi.nlm.nih.gov/books/NBK555956/.
71. World Health Organization, "Urgent Action Needed as Global Diabetes Cases Increase," November 13, 2024, https://www.who.int/news/item/13-11-2024-urgent-action-needed-as-global-diabetes-cases-increase-four-fold-over-past-decades.
72. Center for Disease Control and Prevention, "Prediabetes—Your Chance to Prevent Type 2 Diabetes," December, 30, 2022, https://www.cdc.gov/diabetes/prevention-type-2/prediabetes-prevent-type-2.html?CDC_AAref_Val=https://www.cdc.gov/diabetes/basics/prediabetes.html#.

73. Mayo Clinic, "Trans fat is double trouble for heart health," February 01, 2025, https://www.mayoclinic.org/diseases-conditions/high-blood-cholesterol/in-depth/trans-fat/art-20046114.
74. B Melnik, "Linking diet to acne metabolomics, inflammation, and comedogenesis: an update," Journal of Dermatology, July 15, 2015, https://www.ncbi.nlm.nih.gov/pmc/articles/PMC4507494/.
75. C Martin et al., "The Brain-Gut-Microbiome Axis," National Library of Medicine, April 12, 2018, https://www.ncbi.nlm.nih.gov/pmc/articles/PMC6047317/.
76. B Connizzo et al., "The Detrimental Effects of Systemic Ibuprofen Delivery on Tendon Healing Are Time-Dependent," https://pmc.ncbi.nlm.nih.gov/articles/PMC4079885/#:~:text=In%20addition%2C%20studies%20have%20shown,later%20in%20the%20healing%20process.
77. Dr. John Gannage, "Restoring the Gut Microbiome After Antibiotics." *Markham Integrative Medicine,* Jun 12, 2023, https://integrative-medicine.ca/restoring-the-gut-microbiome-after-antibiotics/#:~:text=Antibiotics%20are%20commonly%20prescribed%20for,syndrome%2C%20and%20chronic%20health%20issues.
78. Cleveland Clinic, "Leaky Gut Syndrome," https://my.clevelandclinic.org/health/diseases/22724-leaky-gut-syndrome.

ABOUT THE AUTHOR

Jeff Bailey is an expert at restoring and maintaining joint health and bone strength. With over 13,000 teaching hours online and in the classroom, he has helped thousands resolve joint pain and return to the activities they love. Working with Jeff, many have avoided joint replacements because of his time-tested method of using the muscles to strengthen joints and bones. In a time where muscle and extreme fitness have stolen the show, Jeff brings a revolutionary approach to health that gets to the problem—arthritis, degeneration, and limited mobility.

At age fifty, Jeff incurred a high-speed ski accident that severely damaged his hip. The turning point came when he realized joints crave compression. Jeff is a trained Rolfer, has appeared on dozens of podcasts, and runs the annual Avita Yoga Teacher Training, which has graduated over one hundred teachers. He leads international retreats and workshops and authored *The Yoga Mind*. Jeff has dedicated his life to helping people live happy, mobile, and independent lives. Now in his sixties, he and countless others are living proof it works. His practical approach to yoga restores and maintains joint health for life.

Explore the Benefits of Avita Yoga!

We use attainable shapes to cleanse and restore your joints and strengthen your bones, resulting in freedom of movement and peace of mind.

Get started today!